The Face-Lift Sourcebook

D0850912

Also by Kimberly A. Henry, M.D.:
The Plastic Surgery Sourcebook
(with Penny S. Heckaman)

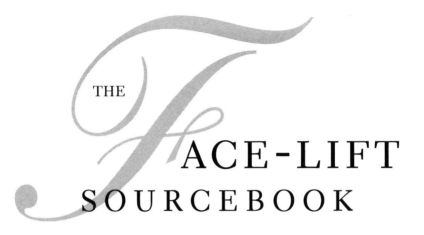

THE FACE-LIFT SOURCEBOOK

Kimberly A. Henry, M.D.

with
Marie Costa

Foreword by
Carolyn J. Cline, M.D., Ph.D.

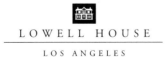

LOWELL HOUSE

LOS ANGELES

NTC/Contemporary Publishing Group

Library of Congress Cataloging-in-Publication Data

Henry, Kimberly A., 1959–
    The face-lift sourcebook / Kimberly A. Henry, with Marie Costa; foreword
    by Carolyn J. Cline.
        p. cm.
    Includes index.
    ISBN 0-7373-0111-2
        1. Facelift. 2. Surgery, Plastic. 3. Face—Surgery. I. Costa, Marie. II. Title.
RD119.5.F33 H46 2000
617.5'20592—dc21   00-057956

Published by Lowell House
A division of NTC/Contemporary Publishing Group, Inc.
4255 West Touhy Avenue, Lincolnwood, Illinois 60712 U.S.A.

Managing Director and Publisher: Jack Artenstein
Executive Editor: Peter Hoffman
Director of Publishing Services: Rena Copperman
Managing Editor: Jama Carter
Interior Design: Robert S. Tinnon Design

International Standard Book Number: 0-7373-0111-2

Printed in the United States of America

00 01 02 03 04 DHD 18 17 16 15 14 13 12 11 10 9 8 7 6 5 4 3 2 1

Contents

Part One: Making the Decision

Foreword

PLASTIC SURGERY: A PSYCHOLOGICAL PERSPECTIVE

If you are contemplating plastic surgery, one of the questions you undoubtedly have on your mind is "Should I really do this?" During more than a decade of private practice as a plastic surgeon, I have found that people can go around and around with this question for days, weeks, months, and even years because the question itself contains many hidden agendas. The major clue to what is going on with this question is the word *should*. What does it really mean? Does it mean "Is it safe?" or "Can I afford it?"

The question that troubles people is "Is it personally, morally, and socially okay for me to do this?" Guilt often lurks beneath the uncertainty. One of my patients confessed, "If I were the person I really should be, I wouldn't have to do this." Another, a graduate student, told me, "My friends will kill me if they find out. They think we should live with what God gave us." (I reminded her that God gave us cosmetic plastic surgeons, too!) Sixty-five-year-old Ann said, "I have the money, but I shouldn't spend it on something so frivolous as a face-lift. I could give the money to my grandson to buy a sports car." (Talk about frivolous!) One gray-haired professor confided, "My mother would roll over in her grave if she knew I was here. I can still hear her voice: 'You're beautiful just the way you are. Stop looking in the mirror all the time; someday a man is going to appreciate you for who you really are.'"

Feelings of guilt have to be resolved before surgery for practical reasons: the unconscious can cause real trouble afterward. "Okay," it says, "you did it. But you shouldn't have, so I'm going to punish you." What kind of punishment? Jessica, a fifty-four-year-old lawyer, experienced unexplained pain after her face-lift. The pain only resolved itself after she acknowledged her ambivalent feelings about not growing old gracefully. Another patient, Pamela, a twenty-five-year-old secretary, could not accept her breast implants as part of herself after having a long-desired breast augmentation procedure. She, too, was only able to accept them after she acknowledged her guilt over competitive feelings with her mother, who had larger breasts. Then there was Margaret, a thirty-eight-year-old nurse, who had diffuse guilt—guilt about being alive. The daughter of a Holocaust victim, her basic philosophy toward life was "It's okay if you do it, just as long as you do not enjoy it." Postoperative depression following her blepharoplasty and breast augmentation sent her into therapy. Later, she wrote me a letter in which she said that having surgery was the best thing she'd ever done. Not only did she love the way she looked, but she had been forced to confront lifelong issues and could finally be happy in life.

Inner Tyrants

These are the voices that hold us back from doing what we want to do, even when we've been intelligent about gathering the pertinent information. These disguised voices of guilt work in devious ways. One forty-year-old woman became absolutely panic stricken just before her breast reduction surgery. Her anxiety was palpable. She was sure she was going to die, so we canceled the surgery. Later, it became clear that she felt she was going against her mother's advice and would therefore be punished. The fact that her mother was long deceased didn't matter. Her mother had always frowned upon doing things for the sake of vanity, and she was still struggling with letting down her mother.

Sometimes a group ethos becomes a tyrant. The woman's movement, a phenomenon in which I participated and regard highly, has spawned a cadre of women who disapprove of plastic surgery intensely. From their point of view, a woman who undergoes such treatment falls prey to the wishes of a patriarchal society, thus internalizing the male gaze. This constricting outlook decreases women's choices and, in fact, becomes a form of tyranny in itself. Berkeley-ites by the droves have come into my office secretly, fearing lest their feminist friends get wind of it. I find this sad. Feminism is about increasing—not decreasing—women's options.

Another tyrannical group ethos uses the word *vanity* in connection with plastic surgery. That's another troublesome and ambiguous word. It is invoked in a pejorative way by those who disapprove of cosmetic surgery. Caring about your clothes, hair, and makeup and exercise is also a form of vanity, but somehow those things are okay. When it comes to surgery, though, vanity is the final bludgeon of the judgmental.

Vanity was believed by the Greeks to be a sister of Beauty and Justice—and a virtue. What happened? Beauty was knocked from her pedestal by the sword of a well-intentioned but now outworn puritanical notion that attention paid to the body took something away from the soul. Those principles are not mutually exclusive.

The idea of symptom replacement is another old saw. As a former psychologist, I remember a strong belief within the profession that wanting to change how one looked through surgery was symptomatic of an unresolved psychological issue, and once the change was achieved something else would replace it as a cause of dissatisfaction. Unfortunately, this misconception survives today.

There is no real difference between cosmetic plastic surgery and reconstructive plastic surgery. We tend to think of the latter as acceptable because it is necessary. Discomfort with a body part that one is born with, or with an aging face that no longer reflects a youthful spirit, is just as deforming to the person who bears it as is a scar from an accident.

Beauty

Whether we like it or not, appearance impacts us greatly. Our fast-paced society allows little time to get to know one another, so a first impression becomes a very powerful factor in making decisions about, say, courting or hiring. Psychological studies show that more attractive people are thought to be nicer, smarter, more competent, and more reliable. Unfair, unfortunately, but true.

Over the fifteen years I've been in practice, the number of men undergoing plastic surgery has increased drastically. I see several interesting aspects to this phenomenon. Men are divorced more often nowadays than in decades past, and are increasingly aware of the tentative nature of the job market even at the highest levels. Men trained to make executive decisions learn quickly to view their physical body image in the context of a "corporate image." Thus it is useful to clarify, streamline, and market them, if you will. Men are simply putting their best foot forward, and their mothers would surely approve of that.

Beauty is a practical issue in our society. When people are uncomfortable with a body part, they feel deformed. And if they feel deformed, they act deformed. They are less assertive, less adventuresome, and sometimes reclusive. Often they settle for less in life, or do strange gymnastics to make a life. Before her rhinoplasty, Barbara would only approach people from a certain angle, lest they see her full profile. Eventually, growing obsessed, she limited not only others' point of view of her, but her own view of things through this angle. After her surgery, she exclaimed, "I had no idea how much time and energy I had bound up with trying to live with the nose I thought ugly. I feel so freed up now and so much more energetic."

Making the Decision

Most people seeking cosmetic surgery are well adjusted. You are probably one of them. But if you have some guilty feelings working in the shadows, you can work with yourself to straighten them out. You can begin by becoming the critical inner voice that is telling you not to do it. Talk out loud. Say all the unspeakable things this voice has been whispering in your ear. Relish the experience. After all, this voice is *you*. Be forceful, say even the ridiculous if it comes into your mind. When you start to hear the voice that wants the surgery, switch to that voice. Vent the yearnings and wishes that voice is expressing. You may find that there is a third voice coming forth, a moderating voice, a deal maker. That is your adult self who wants to negotiate between the other two voices. Speak the thoughts and feelings of the deal maker. Repeat this process a few times. After a while, you will most likely be able to make peace among the warring parties. You may come to realize that the critical voice has been stopping you from doing a number of things in life. Good. You're on your way to positive change. If you can't make peace with yourself, counseling might help. On the whole, I have found that people are very creative deal makers.

You will approach plastic surgery the way you approach most other new situations in your life. One common question people have is "Should I do everything at once or one at a time?" Once the medical safety of any approach is established, the answer depends on your own style and personality. Some people like to dive into the water; others like to put a toe in first and enter gradually. Which type are you? This will give you a clue as to how comfortably you will tolerate surgery.

A fear that many patients have is that once they have plastic surgery they'll never stop, sort of like eating nuts or potato chips. This fear, like most, is groundless. Only once have I encountered a patient with a continual need to change his appearance. And I would not even consider him an addict but rather someone who could not accept himself on a basic level. The vast majority of patients undergo surgery successfully and move on in life with more self-esteem, energy, and determination. As the husband of one of my patients said, "Before her surgery, Jeannie was wishy-washy about making decisions; now she just moves ahead. She even tells me off now and then, which she would never do before. I kinda like it," he said, grinning.

There is such a phenomenon as total body discontent, and that can be solved through psychological work. Joan, a thirty-seven-year-old decorator, was a prime example. She came into my office saying,

"I hate my hips, I hate my thighs, I hate my breasts, I hate my face, I hate all of it." Joan was a poor candidate for plastic surgery. She was disgusted with being overweight and with her unsatisfying life over which she felt little control. She underwent counseling, lost 60 pounds, and emerged with a much more positive self-image. Only then could we surgically address her lack of upper and lower body proportion.

Am I a Good Candidate?

You may be wondering, "How do I know if I am a good candidate for cosmetic plastic surgery?" If you like yourself generally but are bothered by a certain circumscribed area of the body, then it's worth seeking plastic surgery consultation. Once you find that improvement is safe and possible, consider the following questions:

1. *What role do I expect plastic surgery to play in my life?*
   Be sure your expectations are reasonable. Cosmetic surgical change will not bring you a boyfriend or girlfriend if your personality is unpleasant; it won't bring you a job if you are unskilled or unkempt; and it won't keep a wandering spouse close to home.
2. *Have I truly resolved my ambivalent feelings?*
   For instance, do you still hear an invisible voice ringing in your ears saying, "You're so vain, and all this money you're spending, it's a sin." Resolve the conflict by talking with yourself out loud so that you can be 100 percent behind what you're doing.
3. *Have I dealt with the significant others in my life who disapprove of cosmetic surgery?*
   Settle the issue with them, perhaps through the gentle assertion that it's none of their business. You've already settled it for yourself. The last thing you'll want to hear when you're recovering is undermining, guilt-provoking comments from

others. During your postoperative period, you'll need loving care, not criticism.

4. *How will I cope with a complication if I get one?*
Chances are you won't get one. But if you are one of the rare birds who does, you need to be able to say to yourself and mean it: "I will not criticize myself for undergoing this surgery. I went about this procedure thoughtfully and intelligently. That's all I could ask of myself. I'm glad I did it because I really wanted to, and I'll live through this period and be kind and gentle with myself."

Choosing a good doctor is the key to a successful outcome. You need someone who is not only qualified but who really listens to you and cares about you. The first step in finding a good plastic surgeon is to find someone who is board certified or board eligible in the specialty. The American Society of Plastic Surgeons will give you the names of three qualified surgeons in your area. Interview them. Ask to talk to former patients. See if you feel listened to, and trust your reactions. If it doesn't feel right, then this person is not right for you. Move on and find someone who not only does good work but is someone with whom you have a rapport. You will be living with the results of your surgery, not the doctor. Look after your own well-being carefully. If you do, the chances are you will have an extremely rewarding experience.

CAROLYN J. CLINE, M.D., PH.D.

Acknowledgments

WRITING A BOOK IS A DAUNTING PROJECT, and this was no exception. Thanks to my coauthor, Marie Costa, I've also learned that it can be fun. I also thank my children and my staff for their patience and ongoing support.

REGISTERED TRADEMARKS

Autologen® and Dermalogen® are registered trademarks of Collagenesis, Inc.
Zyplast®, Zyderm®, and SoftForm® are registered trademarks of Collagen Aesthetics, Inc.
AlloDerm® is a registered trademark of LifeCell Corporation.
Botox® is a registered trademark of Allergan, Inc.

Introduction

*The purpose of surgery for the aging face is to
allow the individual to live the experience of commuting
between youth and old age in an active and harmonious manner.*
DR. IVO PITANGUY

WHILE IT MAY BE TRUE THAT "you're only as old as you feel," it's hard to feel youthful when you look, well, old. And while everyone ages at a different pace, no one is exempt from the effects of gravity, sun, pollution, and stress—both "good" and "bad." Sooner or later our cheeks and necks begin to sag, our eyelids droop, and wrinkles start to accumulate around our eyes and mouth.

Although some people still insist that it is possible to age gracefully and "naturally," the rest of us welcome whatever help we can find to keep time's ravages at bay. Indeed, in our image-conscious society, we may not be able to afford *not* to do whatever we can to look good for as long as possible. Right or wrong, youth and beauty all too often win out over age and wisdom, so we want to stay young and beautiful (or at least attractive) for as long as we can.

So how do we do that? Good genes certainly help, as can a healthy diet, regular exercise, a good skin care program, and an optimistic outlook. But let's face it, those can take you only so far. Plastic surgery takes up where those self-help programs leave off. Just as growing numbers of people have sought out plastic surgeons to correct what they see as nature's mistakes—whether a bumpy nose, a receding chin, jug handle ears, or undersized breasts—more and more people are turning to plastic surgery to help them keep looking as young as they feel. Often more than mere vanity is at stake, particularly for men, who are showing an increasing interest in face-lifts and other antiaging procedures, not to attract the opposite sex but to maintain a competitive edge in business.

In my previous book, *The Plastic Surgery Sourcebook,* we looked at the whole array of plastic surgery procedures. This book will focus on the face, and specifically on those procedures meant to counteract aging, from the least invasive to the most invasive. We'll start by describing how the face ages, beginning in our twenties and continuing through our sixties and beyond, and then look at the steps we can take to turn back the clock. We'll help you analyze whether and when you need a face-lift, or whether you could benefit from other procedures that are less involved, less expensive, and less disrupting to your life. We'll look at what exactly is involved in each type of procedure, including the costs, what to expect, possible complications, recovery time, and potential benefits. Finally, we'll treat you to the personal journal of a woman who has had a face-lift and gone on to enjoy its benefits.

As a plastic surgeon, I am perhaps more keenly aware than most people of the changes time makes in everyone's face, including my own. I noticed the first signs in my mirror when I was barely past thirty, in the form of baggy upper eyelids and crow's-feet in the corners of my eyes. It didn't take long before I scheduled my first antiaging procedure, an upper lid blepharoplasty. Eventually I went on to have laser resurfacing and Botox injections, with the result that I look not just younger but fresher, more relaxed, and vibrant.

I believe the benefits of age rejuvenation surgery outweigh the risks and are worth every bit of the cost. Hopefully, at the end of our journey together, you will know if the same holds true for you.

Making the Decision

The face is the chief seat of beauty.
LE CAMUS, *Abdeker,* or *The Art of Preserving Beauty,* 1754

CHAPTER ONE

Are You Ready for a Face-Lift?

T HERE IS NO "RIGHT" AGE TO HAVE A FACE-LIFT. Every face is unique, and each of us ages differently and at our own rate. Also, people have widely varying ideas and attitudes about aging. For some, the first hint of a droopy eyelid or a smattering of crow's-feet is a signal that it is time to take action. Others may need a face full of wrinkles and sags before they reach the point of saying, "I need to do something about this."

People often arrive in my office not quite sure that they need plastic surgery but aware that they aren't as happy with their appearance as they used to be. Often the biggest giveaway is that the person's reflection in the mirror looks tired—not old, exactly, just tired, even though the person staring into the mirror feels fine. Another sign is when you're feeling great and other people keep making comments along the lines of "Gee, you're looking a little tired these days. Are you getting enough sleep?" These are indicators that your face is starting to show signs of aging.

Regardless of any clinical signs, the single biggest factor in making the decision to have plastic surgery is how *you* feel about how you look. A sure sign is when you've gotten to the point where every time you look in a mirror your thoughts go something like: "You know, my [eyes, neck, cheeks, forehead, etc.] really, really bugs me. It is not going to get better. If anything it will just keep getting worse. I'm tired of seeing it whenever I look in the mirror, and I am ready to do something about it."

On the other hand, you may not want to wait until you start hating that reflection. Not that long ago, most face-lift patients were in their sixties or older. These days, many people are choosing to have surgery earlier, in their thirties and forties. The advantage is that we can make smaller, more subtle changes that will have long-lasting effects. This approach is closer to preventive maintenance than after-the-fact rejuvenation.

READINESS FACTORS

Plastic surgery isn't like other kinds of medicine. It is totally elective and therefore it must be a choice that the patient is truly ready to make. I don't perform surgery on everyone who comes to me. Sometimes a red flag will go up, and it will be obvious that this person is not a good candidate. Other times the feeling is more subtle. As one of my patient coordinators, Sara Kerbs, puts it, "Dr. Henry, those three things aren't there for that patient." Then I politely tell that person to forget it, at least for now.

The "three things" that Sara is referring to are what I call the three readiness factors: emotional readiness, physical readiness, and financial readiness.

Emotional Readiness

First and foremost, emotional readiness means that having cosmetic surgery feels right to you. This means being certain that it is something you are doing for yourself—not for your spouse, your mother-in-law, or anyone else. Just for you. It also means that you accept full responsibility for making the decision to go ahead with surgery, including making sure that you understand the potential risks as well as the benefits.

It also means understanding that having plastic surgery will not change your life in any significant way. You will still be responsible for paying your bills, going to work, and handling the general business of life. Your "ex" will not return to you just because you've gotten a face-lift or had your love handles suctioned. You will not be assured of that promotion if you get cheek implants or have your eyelids done and your brow lifted.

Emotional readiness also means accepting that it is okay to want to change your appearance. Many people have not yet come to that realization. Despite the huge social emphasis placed on attractiveness, there is also a general attitude that "natural" beauty is the only legitimate kind. It's funny when you think about it, because most people have no problem with wearing braces to straighten their teeth, changing their hairstyle or color, or wearing makeup. And what about all the effort and money we put into losing weight and sculpting our bodies to perfection with exercise and weight training? We get all kinds of positive feedback for taking off that extra 10 or 20 pounds. Our clothes fit better, our attitude improves . . . it's miraculous! Why should getting rid of wrinkles and that tired, saggy look be any different?

When you get right down to it, plastic surgery is an extension of the natural human desire to look as good as we possibly can. When you can honestly say you agree with that statement, then you are emotionally ready to consider having plastic surgery.

Physical Readiness

What does it mean to be physically ready? Plastic surgery may be elective, but it *is* surgery, and any surgical procedure puts added stress on the body. You must be in good enough health that this stress will not lead to complications that could damage the results of surgery, or worse, threaten your well-being. If you have medical problems that might be exacerbated by surgery, you need to discuss them not just with the plastic surgeon but with your regular doctor as well.

In my practice, we start talking about health issues during the initial consultation, including taking a detailed health history, and continue the discussion at the preoperative appointment. I am a physician before I am a plastic surgeon. Much as I would love to operate on everybody who comes to see me and make them feel wonderful about their new looks, I would be doing my patients a big disservice if I did not first make sure they are healthy enough to proceed. I want my patients to be in the best possible health before having surgery, and this is not an area where I am willing to compromise.

Although this is true of all patients, it's especially important for older patients, who are more likely to have a variety of medical problems than are younger adults. Although my patients are all different ages, a significant number are in their sixties and older, and some are in their eighties. A colleague of mine in Marin County once had a patient who was ninety-two! One irony of rejuvenating surgery is that the younger the patient, the less need for aggressive techniques. But the older the patient, the more likely it is that an aggressive approach will cause complications. So the surgeon must carefully tailor the procedure to each patient, taking into account both the changes desired and the patient's health.

Before operating on those patients who are in the upper age ranges or whom I know have preexisting health problems, I make sure that their internists or family doctors are consulted about the procedure. Do they think that it is okay to proceed? How is the patient's blood pressure? What regular medications does the patient take? Are any of these likely to cause problems? For example, blood thinners such as Coumadin or aspirin-containing drugs can pose potential bleeding problems during and after surgery. What about thyroid or other hormonal medications?

So, what can you do to make sure you are as healthy as possible prior to your operation? First, if you do have existing medical problems, it is critical that you let the surgeon know about them as early in the process as possible. This is not a place to be secretive, dismissive, or anything but totally honest and out in the open. Surprises down the road will not be helpful to you or your surgeon.

Second, make sure you follow all preoperative instructions faithfully. If you must vary from them in any way, be sure to let the surgeon know before you go into the operating room. If you get a splitting headache two days before surgery and decide to take an

Advil but neglect to tell your surgeon, you could end up with a hematoma that could affect your final result. You want a perfect result. Your surgeon wants you to have a perfect result. *I* want you to have a perfect result. Withholding information is not in anyone's best interest—especially yours!

This brings to mind something else that is increasingly common, not just in sunny California where I practice but all over the country. Herbal remedies and "natural" supplements. Don't get me wrong here. I think that Eastern and alternative medicine have a lot to offer. The problem is that many so-called natural remedies and supplements contain substances that can affect platelets, the small cells in your bloodstream that enable blood to form a clot. This can lead to bleeding problems, which is why we always tell our patients to stop taking any and all herbs and supplements at least a couple of weeks before surgery.

Just last week I had a patient develop a small yet smoldering hematoma on her right cheek following her face-lift. When we asked her about medications, she swore she had not taken anything prior to her operation except vitamins. We had her bring in the bottles, and one of them was not a vitamin at all but a Chinese herb called ginkgo biloba, which explained her bleeding problem. Eventually she will be fine, but the extra bruising and frequent postoperative visits to our office will make her recovery seem endless. If she had told us ahead of time, we would have postponed her surgery and asked that she not take any of her "vitamins" beforehand.

The same advice applies to alcohol, which can also lead to bleeding. We tell our patients not to drink any alcoholic beverages for at least two weeks before and two weeks after surgery. On the other hand, if you are on medication for high blood pressure, it's important to keep taking it, since uncontrolled blood pressure can also cause complications.

The moral of all this is: 1) Be completely open and honest with your surgeon about your health; and 2) Follow your surgeon's instructions to the letter. After all, it's your health, and your results, that are at stake.

Financial Readiness

Last, or thirdly, as Sara would say, you must be financially ready. I prefer not to discuss financial details with my patients because I want to focus on the patients' needs and on the surgery itself. So instead I have my patient coordinator meet with them to discuss the financial aspects of their proposed procedures.

As you're probably aware, plastic surgery is hardly ever covered by health insurance plans. The only exception is when it is done *primarily* to correct a functional problem, such as an upper lid blepharoplasty to remove skin that is interfering with a patient's vision. This means that in the vast majority of instances the patient pays the full cost of the surgery. This includes not just the surgeon's fee but the fee for the anesthesiologist, if you have one, as well as prescriptions and facility costs if the surgery is done somewhere other than the surgeon's office.

When I was growing up I thought that only movie stars and other rich people could afford something as "frivolous" as plastic surgery. Little did I know how important that "frivolous" option would become in my life, not just as a provider but as a client. (I am a very good plastic surgery customer because I understand its benefits!) Now I know that plastic surgery patients come from all different socioeconomic levels and all walks of life—not just movie stars and models but school teachers, executives, letter carriers, you name it. A recent survey by the American Society of Plastic and Reconstructive Surgeons found that 30 percent of people choosing plastic surgery make less than $30,000 a year, while only a quarter make more than $50,000.

Many practices offer financial assistance to their patients through private financing companies. In our community most people tend to put it on a credit card (a more expensive form of financing, but it works), or pay with a personal check. Sara has told me that she often talks with people who have been saving for years to have a procedure—some of them literally keep their savings under their mattress! Obviously surgery means a lot to these people. It just goes to show that if people feel it is important, they will find a way to pay for it.

Page 218 shows a detailed breakdown of the range of costs for each type of procedure, along with average costs for anesthesiologists and different types of facilities.

WHO IS NOT A CANDIDATE
FOR PLASTIC SURGERY

There are some people who should not have plastic surgery even if they possess all three of the readiness factors described above. Every plastic surgeon should know the warning signs that indicate someone is not a good candidate for plastic surgery. In my practice, I usually see patients several times before I operate on them. This gives me an opportunity to size them up and assess in detail whether they will benefit from plastic surgery and, perhaps more important, how well they will deal with the recovery phase that follows. If I encounter any of the following, I put the brakes on right away.

Indecisive Patients

Some people are reluctant to make the decision to have surgery and want the surgeon to decide for them. When someone asks, "Well, what do you think, Doctor? What do you think I should have?" I explain in detail the operations that I feel would help her. Ultimately, however, it is the patient who has to make—and live with—the decision. If she is unable to do so, I will refuse to operate and tell her flat out that I do not feel she is ready for plastic surgery.

Plastic Surgery Addicts

Some people get "hooked" on plastic surgery. They like the benefits so much that they keep coming back for more—and more, and more. Although it's nice to have our work appreciated, it's also important to know the limitations of what we can achieve. The other type of plastic surgery addict is somehow never satisfied with the results. Regardless of what the surgeon or anyone else thinks, they want to have more surgery to "get it right." This brings us to . . .

People with Unrealistic Expectations

Some patients arrive at the plastic surgeon's office with a "blueprint" or photos of movie stars and say, "Make me look like this." I am cautious with these patients, emphasizing that the goal of plastic surgery is improvement, not perfection. Some surgeons use computer imagery to create before and after photos, with the "after" shot showing the results of simulated surgery. Unfortunately, the real results may not match the simulated ones, thus leading to disappointment.

People Who Think Plastic Surgery Will Change Their Lives

Some patients believe that everything wrong in their lives will suddenly be made right once they get rid of their wrinkles or whatever else is bothering them. In a word, *no!* Following your surgery you will be happier regarding how you look, but underneath you will still be the same person you were before (including all of the same old "life" problems).

People Who Want Plastic Surgery Because Someone Else Wants Them To

An alarm goes off whenever a patient says that her mom wants her to have this, or her boyfriend wants her to have that. As I've said before, you have to want it for yourself, or forget it.

People with Serious Psychological Problems

This includes people who are involved in volatile interpersonal relationships, who have a disturbed or distorted body image, or who want plastic surgery to compensate for other problems such as a fear of dependence or failing health. These patients are definitely not good candidates, either.

People Who Have Recently Suffered a Major Loss

Some patients seek plastic surgery immediately after suffering the death of a loved one, a divorce, the loss of a job, or after their last child leaves home. Surgery should be postponed until after psychological adjustment to the loss takes hold. Sometimes it's not obvious the patient's in crisis until something they say triggers an alarm. For example, a patient may say she doesn't have anyone to take her home after surgery. Or that she doesn't want anyone to know about the operations . . . and by the way she's going through a divorce, or her husband just died four months ago.

Smokers

I've said it before and I'll say it again before we're through. Smoking and plastic surgery don't mix. Many surgeons will refuse to do a face-lift on someone who smokes. At the very least, you have to quit smoking for two weeks before and two weeks after your surgery. So why not quit altogether?

Sometimes you can't exactly pin down the problem, but your instincts tell you that a person is not a good candidate, or at least has some unresolved issues. On the other hand, people can surprise you. I remember one patient who got my psychological antennae twitching. She needed a face-lift, but she didn't like the idea and instead opted to have laser resurfacing on her face and neck. At her initial consultation she complained a lot about her bad back and about a particular chair that we had in the office. I thought she might decide not to go through with it, but she called a few weeks later saying she was ready for the procedure and wanted me to do it.

My initial reaction was "Fine, no problem." It wasn't until her second preoperative appointment that I became a little concerned because she seemed so quiet and withdrawn. When I asked if she had any questions about the procedure she was about to have, she said no. But then she added that I had to do a good job on her because she had "ten friends" who were waiting to see her, and she was a guinea pig for all of them.

Despite some misgivings, we went ahead with the procedure. For five days afterward she was withdrawn, almost hostile. She barely spoke to us when we phoned her to see how she was doing. We were starting to feel we'd made a mistake by giving in to her request. However, a few days later, she had a complete turnabout in personality! She went from being a shy wallflower to a shining star who couldn't wait to show her friends what I had done for her. I loved it. This is what makes my job so exciting: to be able to make people feel fabulous again, to buoy their spirits and restore their self-esteem.

I need to caution you about that last comment, however. Plastic surgery has many benefits, but it will not change your life. What it can do is to make you feel good when you look in the mirror, which will increase your self-confidence and, in turn, make you feel more attractive. You'll seem happier because your eyes will seem brighter. You'll look younger, which can make you feel younger as well. But your problems and all of life's other baggage will still be there for you to deal with. As long as you realize this going in, you'll do just fine.

CHAPTER TWO

Your Aging Face:
The Teens, 20s, 30s,
40s, 50s, 60s, and Beyond

W E'RE ALL FAMILIAR WITH THE visible signs of aging, though most of us don't stop to analyze them in detail. This chapter will look at how aging affects the human face, including the underlying processes that reveal themselves as various wrinkles, droops, and sags. Then we'll take a detailed look at the effects of aging on individual facial areas such as the eyes, jawline, cheeks, and brows.

Let's start with a brief survey of how our face changes through the decades. (See Fig. 2.1.)

THE TEENAGE YEARS

This is the time when the face sheds childish proportions and takes on its adult shape. Few teenagers give any thought to looking old—although many of the habits that they develop during this time will come back later to haunt them. The primary concern of most teenagers is their skin, though no small number seek plastic surgery to change such features as noses, ears, and breasts.

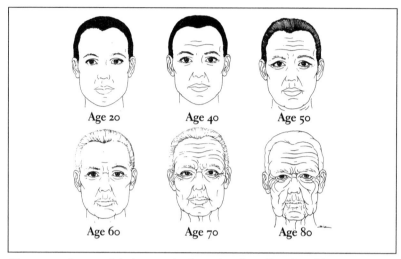

Figure 2.1 Sequential changes in the aging face. Reprinted by permission from *Aesthetic Facial Surgery*, 1995, by Lippincott, Williams & Wilkins.

THE TWENTIES

Ironically, many people in their twenties are concerned not about looking too old but about looking too young to be taken seriously. Their skin is still fresh and firm and nothing has started to sag. Like teenagers, twenty-somethings may indulge in habits such as smoking, drinking, and sun worshiping that will soon begin to show up on their faces. If they have trouble with allergies, they may develop puffiness under their eyes that will worsen with age. Skin treatments (to reduce acne scarring), breast implants, and liposuction are the most popular plastic surgery procedures for people in this age group. (See Fig. 2.2.)

THE THIRTIES

At age thirty, most people have settled into their looks and are pretty happy with their appearance. In fact, if there were an age when we could "freeze-frame" our looks for life, the face we have at thirty

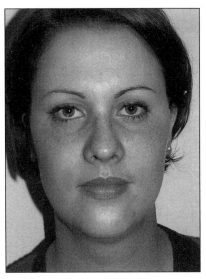

Figure 2.2 Twenty-three-year-old female with beautiful, healthy skin, no wrinkles, and no excess skin.

would be the one most of us would prefer to keep. Unfortunately, it's pretty much downhill from here. As we move into this decade, we might start to notice crow's-feet around our eyes, especially if we have spent a lot of time in the sun, hanging out on the beach, or zipping down slopes on skis or snowboards. Being in the sun a lot also tends to make us squint, as does excess worrying, causing vertical creases to form between our eyebrows.

We may start to notice that our eyes look tired a lot, an effect that is actually due to excess skin on the eyelids—or, in plastic surgeon lingo, upper lid skin redundancy. Still, most plastic surgery performed on people in their early to mid-thirties focuses more on the body than the face. (See Fig. 2.3.) Liposuction and breast augmentation, lifts, or reduction are still the most common procedures during this period.

By age thirty-five, the bloom is definitely off the rose. We don't look quite as fresh and vibrant as we once did. We may look more tired in the morning and at the end of the day due to puffiness around our eyes. The crow's-feet we noticed a few years back are in-

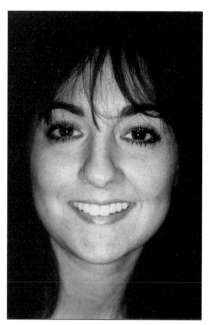

Figure 2.3 Thirty-two-year-old female showing minimal signs of aging.

creasing and getting deeper. Our cheeks start to sag, and creases may become evident on our foreheads and between our eyebrows. Men may also start to see the beginnings of pattern baldness, in the form of a receding hairline or a thin spot on the crown of the head.

By the time we hit our late thirties, the changes have become noticeable. If you are in this age group, you may already be considering such options as Botox injections, collagen injections, lip augmentation, laser resurfacing, even a mini face-lift—or for men, a hair transplant.

THE FORTIES

The forties are when Father Time really starts catching up to most of us, at least in terms of facial aging. For one thing, our foreheads start to develop horizontal creases. In most cases this occurs because of a

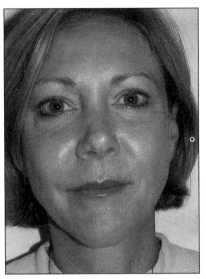

Figure 2.4 Forty-five-year-old female showing minimal signs of aging with upper eyelid skin redundancy, nasolabial folds, minimal wrinkling around upper lip, and slight droop of cheek region.

habit of raising the eyebrows, but some people have so much skin above their upper eyelids by this time that they actually have to raise that skin in order to see. We may also notice deepening vertical creases between our eyebrows, especially if we have neglected to wear sunglasses outside or have a tendency to worry a lot. Our eyebrows start to droop, almost as if the face is starting to close in on itself.

The area around the eyes begins to show puffiness and excess skin, especially for people who have had allergy problems. The crow's-feet that appeared in our early thirties have become deeper and more conspicuous. The middle portion of our cheeks, which started out quite high in our youth, begin to droop, and nasolabial folds become noticeable. (See Fig. 2.4.)

Unless they are quite heavy, the jaws of young people are triangular in shape. As we get older, however, our faces become more square due to sagging skin and fat. The angle of the jawline starts to show the effects of aging anywhere from the mid-thirties to the mid-forties. Generally, the heavier the person, the sooner this is likely to occur.

During the forties, skin texture also becomes noticeably coarser compared to that of a twenty- or thirty-year-old.

THE FIFTIES

The late forties and early fifties is when the neck becomes a matter of concern for many people. In fact, people at this age seem to be troubled more by their neck than any other feature, either by the development of jowls—areas of lax skin and pockets of fat along the lower jaw—or by the loose skin and prominent neck bands known as "turkey neck." Even when it is apparent to me that someone's biggest problems are around the eyes, the patient will tell me that the neck is "what bothers me the most." (See Fig. 2.5.)

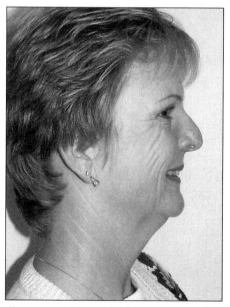

Figure 2.5 Fifty-three-year-old female showing signs of aging around cheek and neck area.

Fine lines will also start to develop on and around our cheeks during our fifties, especially if we are sun worshipers or smokers.

THE SIXTIES AND BEYOND

As we continue to age, jowling around the area of the jawline becomes more prominent and the brows become what we call mortotic: they start to hang down more over the eyes (*totic* means to hang or to droop). This can cause people to look angry or stern regardless of their general mood and personality. The skin is thinner than it was even a decade ago, and wrinkles develop on every part of the face. On people who have spent a lot of time in the sun, the lines become much more noticeable and the skin may have a leathery appearance.

Also around age sixty, the chin and the tip of the nose begin to droop, creating a "witch's chin" and a "plunging tip." Both of these can be corrected with plastic surgery, as can the elongated ears of old age. (See Fig. 2.6.)

The sixties is the decade when many women opt for a face-lift. It is typically the time when people look in the mirror and think, "It's now or never. I've waited this long. I either have to live with what I have or consider doing something about it." By this age, those who decide to have plastic surgery will definitely need a combination of procedures to address most aspects of their face. At this point, people are not trying to look twenty, thirty, or even forty. Instead, they are happy to settle for looking as good as they possibly can.

I once heard a man say he thought it was awful that women wanted to look eighteen at the age of fifty. Obviously this gentleman was unfamiliar with how women really work, or think. Deep down, I think that most women, and men, too, would probably prefer to look younger if they can. Actually, I think men are somewhat biased on this subject because they don't tend to age as quickly as women do. This is partly because a man's facial area, including his neck, has a greater blood supply to the skin in order to nourish his beard. A man's skin is also generally thicker than a woman's. So the effects

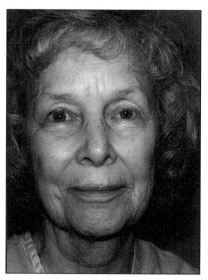

Figure 2.6 Seventy-two-year-old female showing signs of aging around eyes, jowls, and neck area, upper lip wrinkling, and wrinkling of the cheek region.

of aging don't tend to bother them until about age sixty to seventy. That's when men flock to plastic surgeons, saying, "Just cut this off here"—spoken exactly that way. (Sounds like a man, doesn't it?)

IT'S NOT JUST AGE THAT MATTERS: THE EFFECTS OF HEREDITY AND LIFESTYLE

Keep in mind that the above statement is a general progression. Where you fit on the aging face timeline at any given point depends on more, of course, than your chronological age. One of the strongest influences on how quickly or slowly your face ages is your genetic heritage, which determines such characteristics as your general bone structure, the thickness and resiliency of your skin, the size of your pores, and your susceptibility to sunburn or acne. *Intrinsic* aging is something that we have no control over. If your mother and grandmother both had gray hair by age forty, or developed a "turkey neck" by age fifty-five, chances are that you will, too. On the other hand, if your parents are still looking good at age sixty, your odds of looking young longer are enhanced, if not assured.

Intrinsic aging is caused by the skin's gradual thinning and loss of elasticity, as well as by the atrophy, or shrinking, of fat and muscle underneath the skin. The loss of elasticity and shrinking of the underlying tissues cause the skin to sag and become loose. Initially, in our thirties and forties, this appears as bags underneath the eyes. In older people it appears as jowling along the jawline. As the skin thins it also loses its youthful smoothness and begins to feel rougher. Acinic keratoses (*acinic* meaning like a bunch of grapes, *keratoses* meaning horny growths) also become more common, adding to the skin's roughness.

Unlike intrinsic aging, which is the result of time and heredity, *extrinsic* aging is caused by environmental exposure and other factors that can be grouped loosely under the heading *lifestyle*. The effects of extrinsic aging cause the skin to look leathery, yellow, wrinkled, and roughened. The fact is that once you've used up the natural resilience and youthfulness everyone has through the mid-twenties or so, your face starts to show the cumulative effects of your lifestyle. This is especially true if you've spent a lot of time in the sun and/or are a smoker. Under a microscope, extrinsic aging appears as an actual alteration in the structure of the tissue—unhealthy microscopic changes that result from external factors such as sun exposure, smoking, drugs, and stress.

Sun Exposure

Your skin's greatest environmental stressor is ultraviolet radiation from the sun. Even with all the information about skin cancer and early wrinkling, millions of people still spend large portions of their lives playing or working under the sun without using sunblock, hats, or protective clothing. Some people even seek out additional ultraviolet exposure in the form of artificial tanning booths.

Unfortunately, what starts out as a "healthy tan" transforms into something much less desirable as time goes on. We call the effects of long-term sun exposure "photoaging." Among other things, it can cause skin to turn yellow due to a decrease in the number of blood vessels—a natural effect of aging that is aggravated by heavy sun exposure. Alternatively, photodamage can also show up as areas of redness called *telangiectasias* (these can be treated with vascular lasers). Another common result of overexposure to the sun is mottled skin with areas of either hypopigmentation (loss of color), hyperpigmentation (darkened color), or a combination of the two. Such uneven pigmentation can make a person look significantly older than her chronological age. (Figure 2.7, in contrast, shows the results of minimal sun exposure.)

Another hazard of being out in the sun is that unless you are wearing sunglasses, you will have a tendency to squint, which can lead to early and increased wrinkling around the eyes. (See Fig. 2.8.)

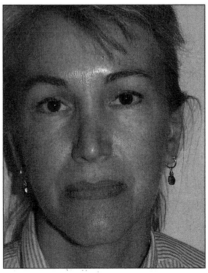

Figure 2.7 Forty-eight-year-old female with minimal wrinkles and minimal sun exposure.

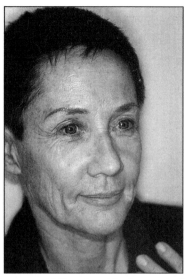

Figure 2.8 Forty-eight-year-old female with deep wrinkles around the eyes, typical of overexposure to the sun.

Smoking

Teenagers take up smoking because they think it makes them look older and more sophisticated. Well, they are certainly right on the first count. If you want to look old fast, try smoking two or three packs of cigarettes a day. Unfortunately, it is a nasty habit that is difficult to break. But I can tell you from personal experience that even some young actresses and models look older than their true age because they smoke.

I can tell instantly when a smoker comes into my office, even if they haven't smoked for two or three years. Besides yellow fingers and teeth, bad breath, and the potential for lung disease or about a dozen kinds of cancer, smoking has a terrible effect on your appearance. Smokers purse their lips a lot, which causes the formation of perpendicular muscle function lines, better known as smoker's lines, around the lips. Also, when people smoke they tend to squint, which contributes to crow's-feet and those vertical creases between the eyebrows. And when they inhale, they suck in their cheeks, which causes creases to form in the cheeks and nasolabial folds. The general quality of their skin is awful, too.

Smoking also causes constriction, or narrowing, of blood vessels including the small vessels under the skin. This means that the skin's blood supply and its access to oxygen and nutrients are severely restricted. This gives the skin a gray, unhealthy cast, even in someone who is otherwise young and good looking. For the same reason, smoking creates a serious risk for any type of plastic surgery, particularly face-lifts. This is because the decreased blood flow can reduce or slow healing or cause the skin to blister and darken. In the worst cases, skin can die and simply slough off.

Secondhand smoke can also be a problem. I had one patient whose entire bridge club took her home after her face-lift. During the early days of her recovery, the bridge ladies smoked up a storm. Needless to say, being enveloped in smoke continuously did not help her healing face and she required some close postoperative follow-up.

Other Factors

Other youth-stealing habits include abusing drugs or alcohol, hard physical work, chronic sleep deprivation, poor diet, and lack of exercise. Yo-yo dieting, with repeated weight gains and losses, also taxes the ability of the skin to return to its original shape.

WHAT CAUSES THE SIGNS OF AGING?

To understand what causes the visible signs of aging, it helps to understand a little bit about the skin and its underlying structures. Though you might not think of it as one, your skin is actually an organ—the largest organ of your body and one of the most remarkable. It serves multiple functions, not the least of which is to form a barrier between you and the outside world while maintaining the integrity of the underlying structures. In other words, it holds all your parts together. Among its other functions are body temperature regulation, immune surveillance, gathering sensory information, and nearly perfect wound healing.

Skin consists of three layers. The outer, visible layer is the epidermis, which actually consists of several thin sublayers, or strata. The surface layer is comprised entirely of dead cells. The other layers contain various kinds of cells that help to protect the body against the environment's harmful effects. These include melanocytes, which produce melanin, a pigment that is thought to protect against the damaging rays of ultraviolet light, and Langerhans cells, which are believed to protect against potential carcinogens and infections. Except for people who have had significant sun exposure, the epidermis does not change significantly with aging. The dead surface cells do, however, tend to slough off more slowly as we age, thus making our skin look tired and older. The purpose of chemical peels, dermabrasion, and laser skin resurfacing (and, to a lesser extent, exfoliants) is to remove these old layers and allow the skin to rejuvenate itself.

Beneath the epidermis lies the dermis, a collagen-rich layer that provides tensile strength and serves as the glue or foundation for a number of embedded structures such as hair follicles and sweat glands. The epidermis and dermis are connected by the basement membrane zone, which serves a critical function in wound healing.

The dermis is considered the most important skin layer; it is where plastic surgeons focus their efforts in trying to prevent or hide the effects of aging. It is composed primarily of two proteins: elastin and collagen. As its name implies, elastin is a rubber-like substance that acts to return the dermis to its normal configuration after an injury. Collagen is a fibrous protein that forms a connective tissue, or framework, that holds the other components of the dermis in place, such as blood and lymph vessels, sweat glands, and hair follicles.

Both collagen and elastin are manufactured by cells called fibroblasts. These little chemical factories also make other important substances such as glycosaminoglycans and glycoproteins. They apparently aid in wound healing, too, though this function is not well understood.

Two other important types of cells found in the dermis are mast cells and dermal macrophages. Mast cells are small cells found mainly near blood vessels in the dermis. They are primarily responsible for inflammation, which is one way the body fights off foreign invasions. Mast cells also play an important role in allergic and hypersensitivity responses.

Dermal macrophages are antigen processing cells. This means that their function is to "seek out and destroy" foreign substances that attempt to enter the body through the skin. Unfortunately, one such foreign substance is injected collagen. The macrophages sense it as an invader and immediately start destroying and removing it, which is why collagen injections don't last very long!

The dermis receives nourishment and oxygen through an abundant array of blood vessels that come up from arteries located in the fat and muscle layers below the skin. These arteries fork off into ever smaller branches, eventually forming a huge network of tiny vessels just underneath the skin. The face and scalp have an especially large blood supply, which is why facial and head wounds bleed so profusely. Men tend to have more blood vessels in their facial (beard) region, which is why they are prone to bleeding complications called hematomas after face-lift surgery. In addition to blood vessels, the dermis contains lymphatic vessels that are responsible for carrying off materials such as fluids and proteins.

Beneath the dermis lies the subcutaneous region, which consists largely of fat. Much as we are conditioned to detest fat, it serves several important functions in the body, one of which is to act as a cushion or shock absorber to protect the skin's underlying structures—muscle and bone.

As we get older, both the epidermis and dermis get thinner. The supply of elastin and collagen in the dermis decreases gradually, and the dermis adheres less well to the underlying tissue. On the surface, these changes result in skin that is looser and less resilient, heals more slowly, and tends to hang from deeper attachments such as along the nasolabial line. At the same time, the subcutaneous fat starts to atrophy, or shrink, along with underlying muscle and bone. The progressive loss of fat and collagen causes any wrinkles or dermal defects (such as depressions in the skin) to look worse.

AGING TOP TO BOTTOM

Let's look at how each part of the face shows the effects of age-related changes in the skin and underlying tissues.

Eyebrow Region

The shape, size, and position of the eyebrows account for much of a face's personality. Eyebrows can also make a face appear more masculine or feminine. (The smooth prominence between the eyebrows is called the glabella; and this region of the face is called the brow-glabella.) On men, the most appealing eyebrow line is one that creates a T-shape with the nose. If the limbs of the T are low, they can be raised with a brow lift. By contrast, a feminine brow is shaped like a Y, with the limbs of the Y lifting up from the nose as opposed to the straight-across masculine line. (This rule of aesthetic proportionality applies to all races and cultural groups.) (See Fig. 2.9.)

Like other parts of the face, the eyebrows tend to droop as we age, which can cause a person to look perpetually worried or angry. Many people seek out brow lifts for this reason — they are tired of always being asked what they are so mad or worried about! A higher brow makes the eye region look more relaxed and youthful, even more elegant and beautiful. Take a close look at some models on the covers of fashion magazines and you'll see what I mean.

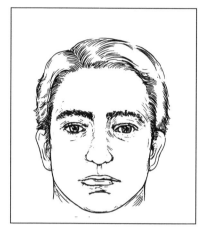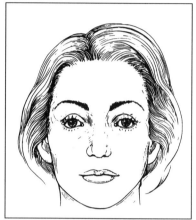

Figure 2.9 Aesthetically pleasing brow-glabella complex in a man with T-shaped configuration and a woman with Y-shaped configuration. Reprinted by permission from *Aesthetic Facial Surgery*, 1995, by Lippincott, Williams & Wilkins.

Eyes

The eyes are usually the first feature to reveal signs of aging. The eyes are also the first thing people notice when they look at your face. This is why blepharoplasty (eyelid lift) is the most popular anti-aging procedure and is often performed on people thirty-five or younger. As early as their late twenties or early thirties, most people begin to show some crepiness around their upper lids. This extra skin makes the eyes look tired, which in turn makes the whole face look tired. Also about this time, the crinkles that show up when we smile may start to linger as crow's-feet even when our smiles fade.

By the late thirties to early forties, the lower eyelids also start to show some bagginess. Around the lower part of the eye, excess fatty tissue known as puffiness can occur at any age—even young teenagers with allergies may show evidence of puffiness. As we age, this area gets worse. A small membrane holds back the fat surrounding the eyeball, and as the membrane ages, it gets thinner until it becomes like tissue paper. As it gets thinner, it loses its ability to hold back the fat, which then becomes much more prominent.

Cheeks

Around the same time the lower eyelids are beginning to age, in the late thirties to early forties, the cheek tissue begins to droop. This creates a groove called a nasolabial line that extends from the corner of the nose, around the mouth, and down around the chin. As the skin and underlying tissue atrophy, gravity causes the skin to hang from its deep attachments. In most people, nasolabial folds first become evident during their forties and fifties. They start earlier and become more prominent in people who smoke or engage in other activities that pucker the mouth.

A person who gains a lot of weight and then loses it will often notice a prominent nasolabial fold. I have also noticed that some body builders who have a very low percentage of body fat and a correspondingly high amount of muscle will develop nasolabial folds at a very young age.

Nose

As we age, the nose grows longer and the tip begins to droop. Most plastic surgeons do not attempt major changes in the shape of the nose after age fifty or so, but minor changes, such as lifting the tip, are common.

Lips

By our late thirties we start to lose fat in our lips, and they begin to shrink, getting progressively thinner and less full as we age. Along with fat, the lips also lose pigment as we get older. Consequently they appear pale and washed out.

People who purse their lips a lot—whether from smoking, sun exposure, or just nervous habit—will develop wrinkled "prune lips." This can start in the late thirties to early forties and continues to worsen into the fifties and beyond. (See Fig. 2.10.)

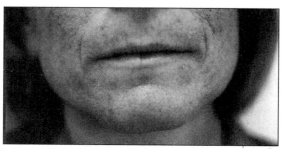

Figure 2.10 Aging of the lips.

Chin

Along with the rest of the face, the chin lengthens as we grow older. It becomes ptotic or takes on the shape known as a witch's chin. Many people also develop "marionette lines"—vertical creases that run from the corners of the mouth down to the jaw. The corners of our mouths may start to droop, causing us to look sad or unhappy.

Earlobes

The ears also enlarge and lengthen as we age. Women who have worn heavy earrings all their lives will develop very long earlobes, which in fact lengthen the entire ear. Droopy earlobes can be corrected during a face-lift, and many patients request this.

Jawline

Another place where age reveals itself is just underneath the chin, where most people eventually develop some laxity, or looseness, of the skin. This happens later in very thin people. Obesity, on the other hand, will mask this excess skin. Instead, heavy people will have a fullness or puffiness under the neck area, which consists of both skin and fat.

Another sign of aging is jowling—excess fat and skin that extends just below the angle of the jawline, near the corners of the chin. This can show up as early as the late forties. Genetically speaking, if your family has a history of developing excess skin or fat under the neck, you probably will, too, unless you have a procedure to correct it.

Neck

Many people who are otherwise untroubled by signs of aging hate what happens to their necks as they get older. The dreaded "turkey gobbler" or "grandmother's neck" is a result of aging of the platysma muscles. These thin muscles run from the corners of the mouth, to the jaw, and down to the collarbone. As we age, the platysma muscles start to separate, giving the appearance of cords running down either side of the neck, with loose skin hanging in between. Some people are unfortunate enough to develop this problem at a very early age. (See Fig. 2.11.)

Acne Scars and Large Pores

Irregularities such as large pores (part of that genetic heritage we can do nothing about) or acne scars (if you missed out on some of the medications currently available to fight acne) can make skin look older. As we age, these areas will continue to look worse. The best treatment for acne scars and/or large pores is some combination of laser resurfacing, small excisional surgeries, dermabrasion, and/or chemical peel.

Wrinkles

Wrinkles are the primary feature that everyone associates with aging. The most common places for wrinkles to appear are on the forehead, around the eyes, on the cheeks, and along the nasolabial

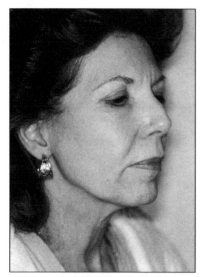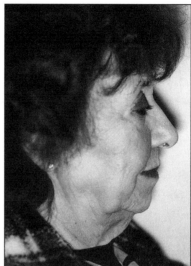

Figure 2.11 Aging of the neck in a fifty-six-year-old female, left, and a female in her seventies, right.

lines. Wrinkles can be categorized into two kinds: fine wrinkes, which can appear all over the face; and coarse or deep wrinkles, which appear most commonly on the forehead and along the nasolabial line.

Deep wrinkles result from changes in the function of the facial muscles and do not disappear when the skin is stretched. By contrast, stretching the skin causes fine wrinkles to fade or disappear. People who have had a lot of sun exposure will develop fine wrinkling all over their faces. I remember a twenty-eight-year-old woman who came to see me for a breast augmentation. She had "sat out in the sun forever"—smeared with baby oil, no less—and had numerous wrinkles. Her skin was actually like that of a woman twenty years older, and despite her youth she was an excellent candidate for a full-face laser resurfacing.

So, what causes wrinkles, anyway? Except for orthostatic wrinkles, which are those natural furrows that are present from birth, facial wrinkles are either *dynamic* or *gravitational*.

Dynamic Wrinkles These develop as a result of repeated right-angle pulling on the skin, which is due to the action of the underlying muscles. As we age, the wrinkles that occur when we smile, frown, wince, or grimace gradually become permanent features. Dynamic wrinkles include those that develop between the eyebrows (called glabellar lines), lines running across the forehead (transverse lines), and around the eyes (crow's-feet).

The more animated a person's face—that is, the more he uses his facial muscles—the more dynamic will be the wrinkles he develops. Back when I was a chemistry major, one of my professors used to comment that I didn't use my facial muscles enough when I spoke. He evidently felt I needed to be more animated. Although at the time my "lack of animation" was largely due to the nervousness I felt around that professor, I am delighted now that I trained myself early on to be careful about not overusing my facial muscles. Today, the number of wrinkles I have as a result of facial function are minimal. Of course my face *does* move (the "wooden look" is not all that appealing, even if it does prevent premature wrinkling), but I'm careful not to overdo facial expressions such as raising my eyebrows. I also wear sunglasses whenever I'm outside in order to avoid squinting—another common cause of wrinkles.

Gravitational Wrinkles In contrast to dynamic wrinkles, gravitational wrinkles develop as a result of the relentless force of gravity pulling our skin toward the earth. Although we may notice gravity's effects sooner on other parts of our bodies such as the buttocks, bellies, and breasts, our faces are not immune, either. As a rule, gravitational wrinkles develop slowly, though some people are affected sooner than others. Gravity is largely responsible for grooves that develop along the nasolabial lines, droopy eyelids, sagging cheeks, and the neck folds referred to as "grandmother's neck" or "turkey neck."

Although aging is inevitable, we don't have to accept its consequences passively. There are techniques to help minimize, or "turn back the clock," regarding just about every aspect of facial aging. So now that we've described what happens to our faces as we age, let's discuss what can be done about it.

CHAPTER THREE

Face-Lift Options in the New Millennium

THE EVOLUTION OF THE FACE-LIFT

Over the course of recorded history, human beings have placed great value on personal appearance. Though standards of what is considered beautiful vary widely among cultures and time periods, and even among individuals, the desire for beauty has remained an unchanging constant. Thus it is no surprise that plastic surgery is one of the oldest branches of surgery, dating back thousands of years. For instance, slaves in ancient Rome occasionally won their freedom and achieved a meteoric rise in fortune. Among other things, their newfound wealth would have enabled them to have any bodily evidence of their former status surgically removed. Other cosmetic procedures performed by Roman physicians included repairing diseased pierced ears, raising slack eyelids, and excising and patching mutilated ears, lips, and noses.

Even in Roman times, plastic surgery was an old practice. The Egyptians had techniques for closing lacerations so that the scars would be inconspicuous, and as far back as 3300 B.C., physicians in ancient India were using forehead skin to reconstruct noses that had been cut off as punishment for adultery. This procedure, developed more than five thousand years ago, is still being used today. Overall, however, plastic surgery evolved slowly and there were few major developments until the nineteenth and twentieth centuries.

Perhaps the most significant event in the evolution of plastic surgery was World War I, when a host of new techniques were developed to cope with the disfiguring wounds of battle. As so often happens, wartime technology spurred the development of methods with broader applications such as repairing nature's "mistakes" and fighting off the effects of aging.

Like the longing for beauty, the desire to stay perpetually youthful dates back many centuries. Chemical peels date as far back as Cleopatra, and surgical face-lifts have been around for several hundred years albeit in a much cruder form than we have today. The modern surgical face-lift goes back at least to the beginning of the twentieth century. In 1901, a German surgeon named Hollander, calling himself a "victim of feminine persuasion," described removing pieces of skin at the hairline and in natural skin folds of a Polish aristocrat in order to "freshen up" her wrinkles and drooping cheeks. In 1931, a surgeon named Lexer reported that he had performed a face-lift on an actress twenty-five years earlier in 1906—decades before any actor started to worry about camera close-ups!

By the mid-1920s, face-lift surgery was becoming increasingly common, particularly in Europe. Published information on the topic, however, was hard to come by. One of the early books on face-lifts and other antiaging techniques was published in 1926 by a Frenchwoman, Dr. Suzanne Noël, who is now considered one of the field's early masters. Her book described procedures for facial plasty, blepharoplasty (eyelid lifts), forehead lifting, and correcting loose neck skin, protruding ears, and loose upper arms. The first before-and-after photographs of face-lift patients were published even earlier, in 1920, by an American doctor named Bettman, who used the same type of incision that is still used (with some modifications) today.

Just as patients once hid—or tried to hide—the fact that they had had plastic surgery, however, most plastic surgeons in earlier decades jealously guarded the secrets of their craft, too. It wasn't until after World War II that plastic surgery came out of the closet, both in terms of public acceptance and in the open dissemination of techniques and procedures. Professional organizations such as the American Society of Plastic and Reconstructive Surgeons (ASPRS) were chartered, and plastic surgeons began publishing regularly in professional journals such as the *Journal of Plastic and Reconstructive Surgery.*

As a result of this continued openness, along with increased research and technological advances, methods have improved greatly, especially during the last few decades. During the 1960s, plastic surgeons turned their attention from the face to the aging neck. They developed techniques for correcting "turkey gobbler" necks and removing excess fat under the chin. The 1970s marked the beginning of the new face-lift era with the development of techniques with odd names (like SKOOG and SMAS) that produced great results. The 1980s introduced liposuction for neck contouring along with new developments in undermining and muscle modifications. The 1990s sparked huge advances in laser technology and the development of endoscopic techniques that reduced the need for large incisions and subsequent scars. And now, at the new millennium, our options continue to expand as the risks decline. Thankfully, the artificial "stretched" look is no longer the only alternative to letting nature take its course!

Along with changes in the field, the last decades have brought about dramatic changes in society, including a major shift in attitudes toward plastic surgery. Once limited to movie stars and wealthy matrons, plastic surgery has become solidly mainstream. Statistics reveal that those who choose to undergo plastic surgery represent a wide spectrum of occupations, ages, and income levels. Although women still comprise the majority of patients, men represent an increasing market segment, particularly when it concerns antiaging procedures such as face-lifts, eyelid lifts, and hair transplants. And both sexes are choosing to have surgery at younger and younger ages. It used to be that most face-lift candidates were somewhere between sixty and seventy years old. Now they are more likely to be in their forties—or even their late thirties. In short, the options for those who want to look as young as they feel are better and safer than they have ever been.

We know now what conspires to make us look old. Our skin gets thinner and loses collagen and elastin plus its firmness, elasticity, and smoothness. Gravity pulls down our eyelids, cheeks, and necks, while the underlying fat and muscle shrink, giving way to various sags and droops. Countless smiles, frowns, and quizzically raised eyebrows wear permanent creases across our foreheads, between our brows, and around our eyes. Fine wrinkles, age spots, and mottled skin offer mute testimony to all the hours and days we've spent working and playing in the sun. In short, our lives are "writ large on our faces," and for many of us, the message is one we'd rather not display.

Fortunately, years of research, trials, and technology have greatly increased and enhanced the arsenal of age-fighting weapons that plastic surgeons now have at their disposal. We can erase fine wrinkles and improve skin quality with lasers, chemicals, and medications. We can excise droopy skin, reposition muscles, remove or add fat, and re-create contour where contour has been lost. We can help people appear more youthful and relaxed yet natural. It may not be as good as being able to hang on to that thirty-year-old face forever, but it's a big improvement over just going along with whatever time and nature dish out.

The technical term for wrinkles is *rhytids,* and the procedure commonly used to remove deep wrinkles is called a rhytidectomy, better known as a face-lift. The face-lift is aimed primarily at correcting droopy skin on the face from the cheeks down. A face-lift alone will not correct droopy eyelids, forehead lines, or lines around the mouth, although procedures to effect these and other improvements can be done at the same time as the face-lift surgery. (These procedures are covered in later chapters.)

As the science and art of face-lift surgery have evolved, techniques have become more complex and individualized. This is good because an approach that produces great results on one patient may not work at all well on another. Face-lifts are as individual and unique as are faces themselves. No one looks precisely like anyone else, with the possible exception of identical twins—and even twins will age differently depending on the circumstances of their lives.

Of course, plastic surgeons also differ from one another and have different treatment approaches to the same problems. Each surgeon has a preferred technique and reasons for doing something a certain way for a particular patient. Thus, if you see six plastic surgeons for a face-lift consultation, you're bound to get six different, but appropriate, approaches to treating your concerns! Nevertheless, they all will (or should) have the same goals—visible correction of the problems both you and the surgeon have identified, naturalness, safety, and ultimately, your satisfaction with the results.

The following sections describe the major face-lift techniques that are used today.

THE BASIC FACE-LIFT

The simplest type of face-lift is a skin lift or skin tightening procedure. This is an improved version of early face-lift operations, in which the surgeon made an incision in the hairline, removed some excess skin, and sutured the incision closed. Since those days, plastic surgeons have refined the process to achieve better, longer-lasting, and more natural-looking results.

To perform this operation, the surgeon makes incisions in front of and behind each ear, extending back into the scalp area. A patient whose problems are limited to the neck area may require just an incision behind each ear. Alternatively, the incisions may be extended up along the hairline above the ears in order to improve wrinkles around the eyes and temple. Even though the incision is made along the hairline, it is usually not necessary to cut or shave any hair before doing a face-lift. Instead, the hair is secured out of the way using rubber bands, clips, or some other method. It's actually a good idea to let your hair grow before having face-lift surgery in order to help hide the incisions while they heal.

To ensure the best possible results, the surgeon will mark your skin prior to surgery so that there is a "map" to follow while making the incisions. The surgeon will also inject local anesthetic into the parts of the face to be worked on before starting the incisions. This helps to reduce bleeding during the procedure and also lessens post-operative discomfort.

After the incisions are made, the skin and subcutaneous tissue are loosened from the underlying muscles using a technique called undermining. Then it is "elevated," or lifted off of the facial muscles in an upward direction toward the cheek area and/or around the neck on both sides. The amount of skin lifted varies, depending on the surgeon. Some surgeons lift the skin all the way to the nasolabial crease, while others are more conservative. The skin is then carefully redraped over the underlying layers, and the wrinkles are removed by smoothing the skin back toward the ears—much the way you would smooth out wrinkles on a tablecloth or sheet. This is where the surgeon's artistic skill comes in. The trick is to remove just the right amount of skin to rejuvenate the face and regain a relaxed, youthful, *natural* appearance. Too little and the results generated are not worth the effort. Too much and you have a face that is flat in the middle and pulled back at the corners of the mouth and eyes—the infamous "wind tunnel" effect that screams "I've had a face-lift."

During the procedure some surgeons remove fatty deposits under the facial skin. Fat may also be removed through a separate small incision under the chin using liposuction or microsuction. The neck platysmal muscles may also be tightened at this point (see Neck Tightening and Contouring on page 47).

Once the redraped skin is in position, the excess skin is cut away and the incision is closed with sutures or staples. (Staples are usually preferable along the hairline because they swell and prevent the tightness that a suture would cause.) The surgeon may also insert thin plastic tubes behind one or both ears to drain away any excess fluids that accumulate after surgery. Finally, dressings are placed over the incision. For my patients, I usually use a head wrap dressing. This is removed, along with the drains, anywhere from one day to a few days after surgery.

A face-lift operation usually takes about three to five hours depending upon the extent of the surgery. The surgery is usually done under either general anesthesia or a combination of local anesthetic and intravenous sedation. Some surgeons perform face-lifts using only local anesthetic, but I don't recommend it. For one thing, it is next to impossible to lie still for that length of time, and a squirmy patient is not easy to work on! Also, if you are under sedation or anesthesia, the experience will be much more pleasant—meaning that you won't remember any of it! So even though having an anesthesiologist may cost an extra $500 to $1,000, this is probably not the type of surgery where you want to skimp on expenses.

Generally, face-lift patients are able to go home a few hours after surgery. It is a good idea to have someone stay with you, at least for the first day or so—a friend, a relative, or even a professional nurse. Alternatively, some facilities provide overnight care. Many areas also have special recovery centers or retreats that cater to plastic surgery patients.

You will need to sleep with your head elevated for a week after the surgery in order to keep swelling down around the facial area. Most patients experience mild or moderate pain following a face-lift, and this can be alleviated with prescription pain medication. The main discomfort associated with face-lifts is a feeling of tightness around the neck area. This lasts for two or three weeks and then gradually improves over the next several months.

SMAS and Composite Face-Lifts

Unfortunately, having a face-lift doesn't stop the aging process. It just sets the clock back a few years. Some surgeons have tried to address this problem by going deeper and manipulating subcutaneous tissues in addition to the skin itself. Just underneath the fatty layer of the face, covering the muscles, is a thin layer of tissue called the superficial musculoaponeurotic system, or SMAS. In an SMAS face-lift, this tissue is pulled up and tightened along with the skin. A composite (or deep plane) face-lift goes even deeper, tightening all the layers of facial tissue down to the bone. (See Fig. 3.1.)

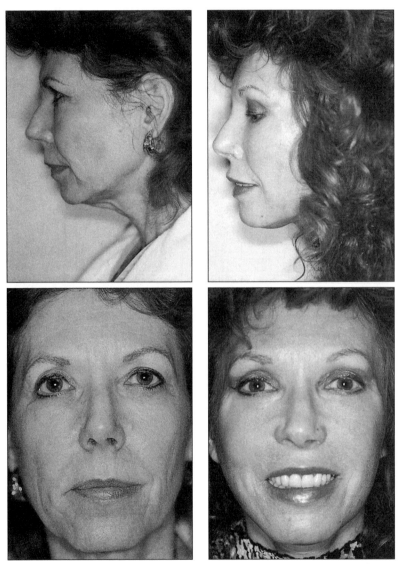

Figure 3.1 Fifty-six-year-old female before and eight days following full-face laser, face-lift with SMAS dissection, brow lift, and upper and lower lid blepharoplasty. Note that the patient still has some swelling under the chin and is continuing to go through the healing process with the laser resurfacing of her skin. *Top,* side view before and after. *Bottom,* front view before and after. *Top of next page,* three-quarter view before and after.

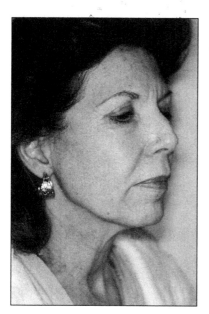 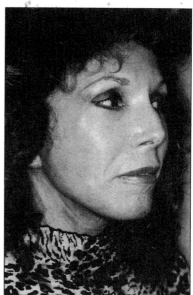

The primary goal of SMAS and composite face-lifts is to make the results last longer. Whether they actually do is a matter of debate. In any case, these types of face-lifts are controversial, mainly because of the increased risk to the patient. Some surgeons perform them as a matter of course. Others refuse to do them at all out of concern that they could injure the facial nerves (which are exposed during surgery) or other facial structures. Some surgeons also believe that the suturing techniques required for deeper face-lifts result in a less natural appearance, especially with animation.

The recovery time for SMAS and composite deeper face-lifts is longer than for a skin lift—in some cases considerably so. A small percentage of patients experience some temporary facial paralysis, and in a very small percentage the paralysis is permanent. If you do opt for an SMAS or composite face-lift, make sure your surgeon has experience with the procedure and is extremely meticulous and careful before going ahead. (See Fig. 3.2.)

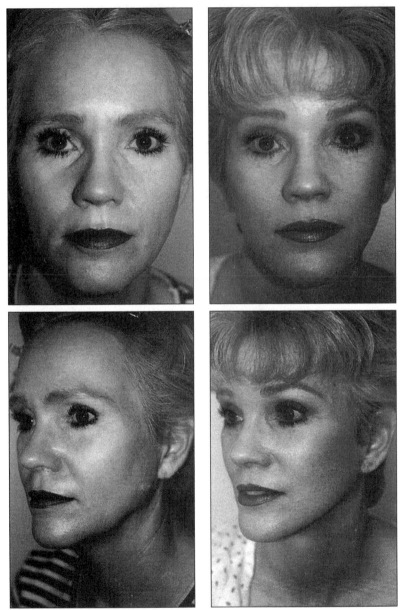

Figure 3.2 Full-face rejuvenation and crow's-feet correction with SMAS face-lift, forehead lift, neck lift, and eye lifts. (See also top of next page.)

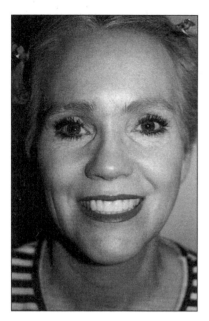 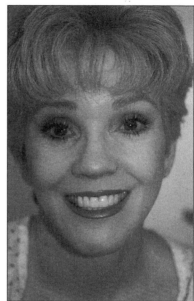

Hamra's Face-Lift

The term *composite face-lift* is also used to describe a technique developed by Dr. Sam Hamra, a plastic surgeon in Texas. Dr. Hamra believes that because the entire face ages together, the entire face should be dealt with at once. His operation consists of a forehead brow lift, upper and lower lid blepharoplasty, cheek internal suspension, and tightening of the neck platysmal muscle (these procedures are covered in chapters 5 and 6), along with a lower face-lift in the deeper SMAS layer, all performed at the same time. The entire procedure takes most surgeons six to eight hours to complete.

Hoefflin's Face-Lift

Steve Hoefflin is the "plastic surgeon to the stars." He has worked on numerous celebrities and gets good results for the most part (but then his patients were all great looking to start with). Among his accomplishments is Michael Jackson's nose, which, according to the surgeon, is exactly what the star wanted.

Dr. Hoefflin developed a face-lift technique in which the skin and subcutaneous tissue are completely released off the face and then stretched back over it, after which the excess skin is removed. If necessary, excess fat underneath the skin is trimmed, and in some patients fibrous bands near the mouth are also released. The technique is relatively simple to perform, and the risk of nerve injury is much less than with the SMAS or composite approach.

Mini Face-Lift

Many women come to see me while still in their middle thirties to early forties. They are beginning to see signs of aging, especially under their jaws and in their cheeks, and are unhappy about it but not ready for a full face-lift. For these people, a mini face-lift is a good option.

For this procedure, the surgeon makes a small incision in front of the ear, then lifts a small area of skin. The skin is undermined and pulled back, the excess trimmed away, and the incision closed. It is called a mini face-lift because the incision is much smaller than in a regular face-lift. To get the full benefits of this procedure, you need to be on the youngish side—generally no more than forty-five.

A mini face-lift can be performed under local anesthetic. The recovery time is shorter than that for a full face-lift (about four or five days).

FINE-TUNING THE FACE-LIFT

Often the difference between a good face-lift and a great one is a matter of paying attention to details, such as the following:

Neck Tightening and Contouring

Many people who are otherwise untroubled by the effects of aging will nonetheless confess that they hate their necks. One common problem is the "turkey neck" or "grandmother's neck." This happens because as we age, the platysmal muscles—which run from the corners of the mouth to the jaw and down the sides of the neck to the collarbone—start to separate, giving the appearance of two bands extending the length of the neck with loose skin in between. Tightening these muscles is often done in combination with a face-lift. This procedure is called an anterior platysmaplasty.

A number of different techniques can be used to tighten the platysma. These include suturing it together, transecting and removing part of it, or cinching it up like a corset. Some surgeons even suspend two or three strands of sutures across the neck, similar to a purse string held taut, which gives a nice, defined angle to the jaw. (See Fig. 3.3.)

If done in combination with an SMAS lift, platysmaplasty is usually done right after tightening the SMAS layer in the cheek region.

Neck tightening and contouring are discussed in more detail in chapter 5.

Submandibular Glands

Sometimes an otherwise perfect face-lift can be marred by an unexpected fullness that remains just under the jawline. One cause of this problem can be the submandibular glands, which sit right underneath the jawbone. If this is detected ahead of time, the surgeon can remove a portion of the glands during the face-lift procedure. Sometimes tightening the platysma can help improve ptotic or droopy submandibular glands, but this effect may be only temporary. In these cases repeat exploration and removal may be necessary.

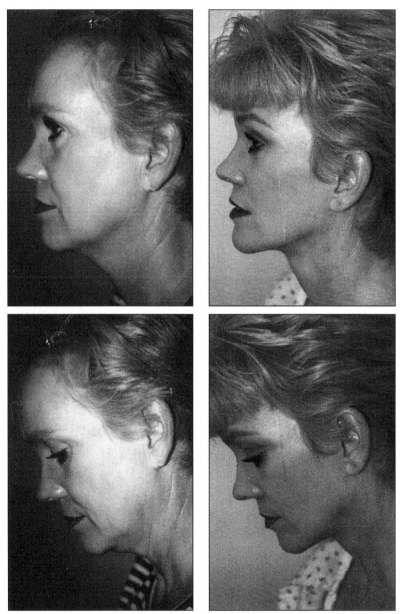

Figure 3.3 *Top, left and right,* platysmaplasty (neck muscle tightening). *Bottom, left and right,* transposition flap (tucks neck when patient looks down).

The Digastric Muscles

Another cause of unwanted postoperative fullness is bulkier-than-usual anterior digastric muscles. These muscles look like two bands that radiate out from just underneath the chin. Sometimes they are hidden by fat and reveal themselves when the fat is removed during the face-lift. To correct this problem the surgeon will need to remove them.

AUGMENTING A FACE-LIFT

More often than not, once patients have decided to have a face-lift, they will ask me, "Well, Doctor, since I'll already be under anesthesia (and since I'm already investing all this time and money), is there anything else you think I might need to have done?" Often this question will come up shortly before the patient is scheduled to have surgery.

By this time it should be apparent that a face-lift alone may not be enough to give your face the more youthful look you desire. There are, however, a number of other procedures that can be done simultaneously with, or following, a face-lift to greatly improve the results. (See Table 3.1.) One reason you may want to think about some of these other procedures is to keep your face from looking as though you are several different ages at once. For example, a firm, youthful neck can make your droopy eyelids or brows look even older by comparison.

TABLE 3.1 Surgical and nonsurgical procedures that can be performed simultaneously (with chapter references for details).

Nonsurgical Procedures (Chapter 4)

- Collagen or Botox injections to increase fullness or reduce wrinkles
- Soft implants to reduce wrinkles and augment facial features
- Fat injections to erase wrinkles and "plump up" shrunken facial areas
- Cosmetic tattoos such as permanent eyeliner and/or lip liner

Surgical Procedures for the Lower Face (Chapter 5)

- Cheek lifts or implants to restore healthy fullness to the cheeks and/or reduce under-eye puffiness and nasolabial lines
- Chin implants to give more definition to the chin and jaw
- Jaw recontouring
- Liposuction or microsuction to contour the neck and jaw
- Lip augmentation to restore youthful fullness to the lips

Surgical Procedures for the Upper Face and Eyes (Chapter 6)

- Forehead or brow lifts to correct forehead creases and/or droopy brows
- Blepharoplasty (eyelid lifts) to correct droopy eyelids or under-eye puffiness
- Forehead recontouring

Skin Resurfacing (Chapter 7)

- Laser resurfacing to remove surface wrinkles and discoloration such as age spots

CHAPTER FOUR

Nonsurgical Options

L ET'S FACE IT, IF SURGERY IS NOT A REQUIREMENT—to remove a
cranky gallbladder or an infected appendix, for instance—why
would you even consider going "under the knife?" Well, until about
fifteen or twenty years ago, most people would have said, "Forget it.
Not interested." Unless you were a victim of burns or other deforming injuries, wanting to have plastic surgery meant you were
superficial, vain, or had major psychological problems!

Not any more. Since the 1980s, attitudes toward plastic surgery
have undergone a dramatic shift, particularly among the generation
born since World War II. This is not all that surprising when you
think about it. After all, people have been altering their bodies for
aesthetic reasons for millennia. Some African tribes, for example,
still practice customs such as decorative facial scarring, wearing
neck bands to elongate their necks, or using special instruments to
lengthen their earlobes. When you think about it, there's not a
whole lot of difference between those so-called primitive customs
and such "modern" practices as dyeing hair, wearing artificial nails,
using braces to straighten teeth, or "sculpting" your body through
daily workouts. If you regard these approaches as understandable
and normal, cosmetic surgery is a logical next step.

As I pointed out in chapter 2, if most of us could just keep the
faces we had at age thirty, we'd be perfectly happy. Since that's not
possible, most people would just like to look as good as they can for
their age, and if that means plastic surgery, then it's okay with them.
Still, many people are reluctant to take what they see as the drastic

step of a face-lift. I can't tell you how many times I have heard the refrain "I don't want a face-lift, Doctor, just get rid of _____." (Fill in the blank: "this turkey neck," "these crow's-feet," "this double chin," "these puffy eyes," etc.)

Fortunately there are other less invasive and less expensive procedures that can achieve results that, though they may not be as dramatic, are nonetheless pleasing and worthwhile. And none of them exclude the possibility of having a face-lift later should you decide to go on to the next level. On the other hand, if you decide you do want to go ahead with a face-lift now, you may want to do one or more of these procedures at the same time, in order to achieve the best possible results.

This chapter focuses on nonsurgical alternatives for rejuvenating the aging face, including:

- Injectable implants including collagen, Autologen, Dermalogen, and fat injections
- Botox injections
- Soft implants including SoftForm and AlloDerm
- Cosmetic tattoos

Chapters 5 and 6 will look at various surgical options that can be done in addition to or instead of a face-lift, and chapter 7 will discuss skin resurfacing procedures with an emphasis on laser techniques.

INJECTABLE IMPLANTS

Among the least invasive—and most temporary—methods of facial rejuvenation are injectable implants including collagen, Autologen, Dermalogen, and fat injections. They are also extremely popular: The American Academy of Cosmetic Surgery reports that 323,000 injectable implant procedures for soft-tissue augmentation were performed in 1996. That number is expected to grow by about 7 percent a year through at least 2003.

Injectable implants are great for erasing or reducing wrinkles such as the lines that form around the lips of smokers, crow's-feet, nasolabial creases, and the "worry lines" that form on the forehead or between the eyebrows. They can also help to reduce or erase depressed scars such as those caused by acne. And last but far from least, they are commonly used to augment lips, not just in older people whose lips have gotten smaller as they've gotten older, but in young people who want the sexy, pouting look of full lips made popular by models and actresses.

Collagen

Collagen, remember, is the connective tissue that is made by cells in the dermis, which helps give our skin its strength and firmness. As we age, our bodies produce less collagen and our faces start to develop various lines and depressions, not to mention shrinking lips. Collagen injections use a synthetic collagen to replace what has been lost through the aging process. Injecting collagen under the skin adds bulk and firmness to the tissue. The procedure is simple, relatively inexpensive, and increasingly popular. (In our office, you can always tell when high school reunion season has rolled around by the number of collagen syringes lined up on the counter, ready to smooth out and "plump up" our patients prior to the big event!)

The collagen used for most cosmetic injections is a synthetic form developed from bovine collagen—i.e., cow skin. Most people tolerate bovine collagen very well, but a few will have an allergic reaction. For this reason, it is necessary to perform a skin test prior to beginning collagen therapy. The test consists of injecting a small amount of collagen under the skin of your inner arm, then observing it over a period of three weeks. If you do not develop a red bump or rash at the injection site, the test is considered negative and the doctor can begin the injections. If the area is red, itchy, or swollen, the skin test is considered positive and collagen injections should not be used. This is more likely to happen in people with a sensitivity to beef or other cow products. Collagen should also not be used in pregnant women or people who suffer from autoimmune diseases such as rheumatoid arthritis or lupus.

To perform the procedure, the surgeon simply injects tiny amounts of collagen along the wrinkles or in numerous sites on the lips. Synthetic collagen compounds contain a local anesthetic such as lidocaine to help numb the injection areas. The procedure is pretty uncomfortable, however, though most people tolerate it without much difficulty. When doing lips, some surgeons use a local anesthetic to numb the entire lip area before injecting the collagen. Following the injections, the area will be swollen and may be slightly bruised as well. The swelling starts diminishing generally within sixteen to twenty-four hours.

The number of syringes needed for a collagen treatment varies depending on the number and severity of the wrinkles being treated and/or the lip size desired. Most patients require between 1 and 2 cc of collagen. All collagen used in this country comes from a single source, Collagen Aesthetics, Inc. (formerly Collagen Corporation), a company based in Palo Alto, California. It is sold under several different brand names such as Zyplast and Zyderm, and costs around $375 to $425 for a 1 cc syringe.

Collagen's main drawback is its impermanence. The body will eventually absorb all of the synthetic collagen and the procedure will have to be repeated, sometimes as often as every two or three months. For this reason, and because of the risk of allergic reactions, a fair amount of research in recent years has focused on finding alternatives to bovine collagen. Two of the hottest items to come on the market lately are Autologen and Dermalogen, both of which are made by a biomaterials company called Collagenesis, Inc.

Autologen

Autologen is an injectable collagen implant derived from the patient's own skin using a process patented by Collagenesis, Inc. To produce it, a small amount of skin is "harvested" from your body. This is easily done during a face-lift, tummy tuck, or other surgery where skin is already being removed, but the surgeon can also simply take some skin from an area like your inner thigh in a separate procedure. The skin is frozen and sent to the company's laboratories where it is processed into a collagen-rich dispersion and put into preloaded syringes. The processing takes four to six weeks, after which a simple phone call is then all that is needed to have syringes of your own collagen shipped directly to your doctor's office overnight. For best results, Collagenesis recommends three Autologen treatments over a period of six to eight weeks.

The skin at the injection sites may be red for about forty-eight hours after the injections, and some patients develop bruises that can take a few weeks to heal. Since Autologen is made from your own skin, however, the chances of an allergic reaction to it are practically nil. Even better, it should last longer than animal-derived collagen — a lot longer, according to Collagenesis. The company claims that patients have shown 75 percent or better correction lasting over a year after final treatments, and some patients have experienced improvements lasting three or more years.

The cost for Autologen ranges anywhere from $750 to $1,500 for two to three syringes. If you are having skin removed for another procedure but don't want to use Autologen right away, the company will store unprocessed tissue for up to five years for a nominal annual fee.

Dermalogen

Like Autologen, Dermalogen is derived from human skin, but in this case the skin comes from human cadavers by way of tissue banks that provide donor skin to hospital burn units. (If that thought makes you nervous, you should realize that the risk of disease transmission from human-donated tissue is virtually zero. Tissue banks are strictly regulated by the government and overseen by the American Association of Tissue Banks. This ensures that all donors are

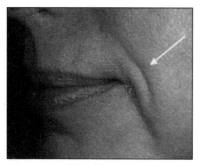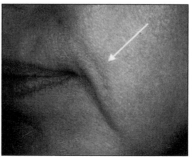

Photo Courtesy of Dermalogen Corp.

Figure 4.1 Wrinkles injected with Dermalogen (before and after).

carefully screened and tested to reduce the risk of disease transmission. In addition to burn surgery, donor tissue is also used for periodontal [gum] surgery and bone implants. Hundreds of thousands of people receive such implants every year.)

According to Collagenesis, Dermalogen is superior to bovine collagen because it contains intact collagen fibrils, an elastic network, and proteoglycans similar to those found in the skin's dermal layer while bovine collagen contains digested cow collagen in small segments. The jury is still out on how much longer it lasts, however. In my practice, patients are opting more and more for Dermalogen over bovine collagen because it does appear to last longer. We administer the treatments in three stages over a six-week period. The first week we inject anywhere from 1 to 3 cc of Dermalogen. Two weeks later we do a second treatment using the same amounts, and two weeks after that we repeat the treatment again. Layering the Dermalogen appears to make it last longer. (See Fig. 4.1.)

The injection process and aftereffects are similar to bovine collagen or Autologen. However, because Dermalogen does not contain any local anesthetic, the injections are more painful. As with Autologen, the skin may turn red or blanched (whitened) at the injection sites for a couple of days, and there may be some bruising as well.

Fat Injections

As we've learned, gradual loss of fat is one of the factors that contributes to facial aging. The concept of injecting fat to erase lines and plump up shrunken facial areas such as the cheeks, forehead, and eyes has been around for a few decades. It was treated with skepticism until quite recently, however, and many surgeons believed that it didn't work. In the mid-1990s, Dr. Sydney Coleman, a New York–based plastic surgeon, reintroduced the idea with some important enhancements. Using a very specific technique and administering the injections over multiple sessions, Dr. Coleman has achieved some remarkable results. I attended one of his seminars several years ago. For his presentation, Dr. Coleman introduced an unusual twist. Instead of showing the before pictures first, followed by the after pictures, he would display a photo of a youthful, nice-looking individual, followed by a drawn, emaciated version of the same person prior to the series of injections. The reverse presentation made the impact of the improvements that much more dramatic. These people looked great!

A fat injection is actually a tissue graft of sorts in which you act as your own donor. The surgeon takes fat from one part of your body such as your inner thigh, stomach, or love handles, and re-injects it in the areas to be enhanced such as your lips or the wrinkles on your cheeks, chin, or around your eyes. It can even be used to fill out aging hands and hide those prominent veins that become increasingly unsightly as we get older. (See Fig. 4.2.)

For this procedure the donor site is numbed with local anesthetic, and then the fat is withdrawn using a syringe and a cannula. Lest you get too excited about the prospect of moving fat from where it is not wanted to where it is, be forewarned—this is not liposuction. Only a small amount of fat—usually about a third of an ounce, or 10 cc—is all that is needed to take care of a face full of wrinkles *and* enhance the lips.

Once the donor fat is obtained, the area to be built up is numbed

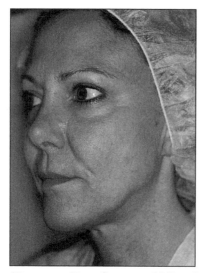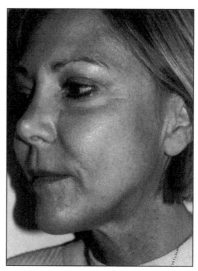

Figure 4.2 Forty-five-year-old female with fat injection to the nasolabial folds and cheek regions (before and after). Notice the more youthful appearance following the procedure.

and the fat is re-injected in a thin layer under the skin. Though Dr. Coleman claims his technique is superior (he centrifuges the fat and drains off all fluid before re-injecting it), other surgeons inject the fat immediately after obtaining it from the donor site using the same syringe and changing only the needle in between. The procedure is straightforward and the discomfort minimal. Since the fat injected is the patient's own tissue, there is no risk of an allergic reaction. Patients can usually return to work a few days after fat injections, and sometimes sooner. Since a good portion of the fat injected in any one session will be reabsorbed by the body, most surgeons recommend doing three or more treatments over several months.

Fat injections last longer than any of the collagen products, though how long is not known. Some doctors claim that the fat that "takes"—that is, which doesn't get reabsorbed within the first six weeks or so after surgery—will stay in place for many years. One key may be in handling the fat as gently as possible during the procedure in order to keep the fat cells intact. As with Dermalogen, having several treatments over a period of time and layering the fat seems to give longer-lasting results.

We have administered fat injections to several patients with terrific results. One of my office assistants had prominent nasolabial folds and deep crevices around her cheeks. In a forty-five-minute operation under straight local anesthetic, I removed a small amount of fat from her hip and reinjected it into her face. We also injected more fat than was actually needed in order to allow for tissue reabsorption. As of this writing, about a year after the procedure, she still has almost complete elimination of the nasolabial folds and considerable improvement of her cheek crevices.

BOTOX INJECTIONS

Botox is an extremely diluted form of *botulinuum* toxin, the same chemical that causes botulism, a lethal type of food poisoning. The toxin acts by blocking nerve impulses from the brain that tells muscles to contract. When it is ingested this action causes system-wide paralysis and, in most cases, death. But as is so often the case in medicine, a substance that is poisonous in some circumstances can be beneficial in others (examples include curare, which is used in anesthesia, and chemotherapy, which uses poisons to kill ravaging cancer cells). The same holds true for the botulinuum toxin. When a very tiny amount is injected into a muscle, the result is temporary weakening or paralysis at the injection site. This makes it very useful in situations where muscle contractions are causing problems, such as muscle spasms.

Botox was initially developed in the 1980s as a treatment for problems affecting the eye muscles such as blepharospasm, a condition in which the eyelid muscles contract involuntarily. At the least blephpharospasm causes the eyelids to twitch. At its worst it can cause them to lock shut, making a person functionally blind. Injecting Botox causes the eyelid muscles to relax, thus ending the spasms. The idea of using Botox to relax wrinkles was reportedly developed by a Canadian ophthalmologist. Presumably she had observed that

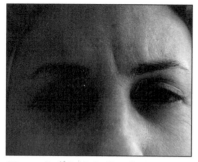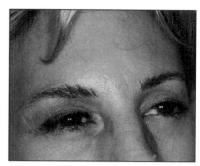

Figure 4.3 *Left,* before botox injections to the glabellar area (between the eyebrows). *Right,* after injections. Notice the loss of wrinkle formation even when the patient is trying hard to frown.

patients injected with Botox not only regained control of their eyelids but looked noticeably younger as well. (See Fig. 4.3.)

Since Botox acts to weaken muscles it is used to treat dynamic wrinkles—those caused by overuse of facial muscles. It is especially effective on the corrugator and procerus muscles, which are responsible for the worry lines between our eyebrows and forehead creases. It is also good for reducing or erasing crow's-feet and lines around the upper lip. As a bonus, when injected around the upper lip Botox causes it to appear a bit fuller (the mechanism of this is not clear). Botox can also be used to improve lines or muscle bands on the neck. Some surgeons use Botox to pretreat facial areas prior to other procedures, such as laser resurfacing, on the theory that patients can have better results if their skin is not being subjected to muscle overactivity during the healing process.

A Botox treatment consists of a series of injections along the target muscles. Most patients do relatively well with the injections and experience only minor discomfort. Occasionally a patient has a headache following the injections, but again this is mild and treated easily using an over-the-counter pain reliever. A typical treatment costs $500 to $750.

The effects of Botox take anywhere from a few hours to several days to become apparent and begin to wear off within a couple of months. This means that the injections must be repeated every three to five months. After several treatments, the effects may start to last longer, sometimes as long as six or eight months. It is thought that with repeat injections a muscle will become so weak that it will lose total function.

When I had my first Botox injection, I could see immediate results the first day. By the end of the week, I could not wrinkle my forehead or make a mean face, and my face looked much smoother and more relaxed. My office manager, who also had the injection, said she felt like her skin had been smoothed out or stretched. She thinks that she looks much more serene. I have Botox injections perhaps every three to four months, which is pretty typical. On the other hand, my office manager has gone almost nine months without needing a repeat treatment.

Complications and Side Effects

The manufacturer maintains that there are no complications from the use of Botox, even though it is a toxin. This is because (1) the amounts used are extremely small, being measured in billionths of a gram; and (2) it remains localized at the injection site and does not spread through the body. However, since any site that is injected with Botox will eventually weaken, it makes sense to be very careful about the location of the injections. For example, after one of my injections my right upper eyelid started to droop, a condition called ptosis. It stayed that way for almost three days. If this should happen to you, be assured that the ptotic eyelid will return to normal. Mine did and I've had several injections since with no problems.

SOFT IMPLANTS

If you don't want the expense and bother of repeated injections, soft implants offer a long-lasting alternative. The two main types are

SoftForm, a synthetic implant, and AlloDerm, which, like Dermalogen, is made from donated human skin. Unlike collagen, these
are permanent implants that do not reabsorb or disappear after being put in place, though furrows may reappear slowly over time.
Both types are ideal for patients who do not want to go through
more elaborate procedures that require time off from work and
greater expense.

SoftForm

SoftForm implants consist of strands of soft, thin tubing made from
a polymer called ePTFE (expanded polytetrafluoroethylene), otherwise known as Gore-Tex—the same material that revolutionized
the outerwear apparel industry. In addition to being waterproof and
"breathable," ePTFE is biocompatible, meaning that it can be used
inside the body with no ill effects. It has been used in medical applications, including blood vessel and hernia repair, for more than
twenty years. (See Fig. 4.4.)

Because it is microporous (has many tiny pores), SoftForm allows
for tissue ingrowth without the formation of typical scar tissue en-
capsulation. This permits the body to incorporate it in a more natural way than with less porous implants. On the other hand,
because it does not degrade or change its form after implantation,
it can be removed easily if necessary because of infection or other
problems.

SoftForm works by providing support and structure underneath
the skin. It essentially reduces the depths of creases or furrows by
raising them to the level of the surrounding skin. The implants can
be used to improve nasolabial folds, forehead lines, frown lines, and
marionette lines (creases that go from the corner of the mouth onto
the chin), as well as to enhance noses, chins, cheeks, and lips. In
some cases it may be necessary to use additional filler such as collagen or fat to achieve full correction.

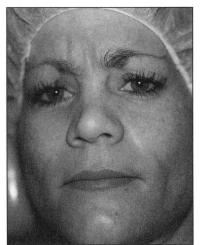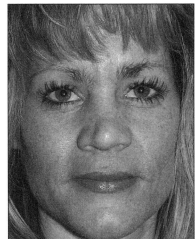

Figure 4.4 SoftForm to lips and glabellar area (before and after).

To use the implants, the surgeon threads one or more strands underneath the skin in the area to be enhanced. The procedure is very easy to do, takes about thirty minutes, and can be performed under local anesthesia. A few small incisions are required to place the material correctly. The sutures are removed about three to five days after the procedure. There may be some swelling or bruising that lasts for a few days; these can be covered easily with makeup. There may also be a sensation of tightness in the treated area for a week or so. Most patients return to normal activities the day after treatment.

Although the results of the implants are apparent immediately or soon after surgery, full healing takes three to four months. Within five to seven days most people will not be able to tell that you have had a procedure. Scarring is rare, except for tiny scars at the incision sites, which are located where they will be largely unnoticeable. Patients will always be able to feel the implant under the skin, although this lessens over time.

No allergies to ePTFE have been reported. While it is possible to have an allergic reaction to almost any material, SoftForm implants are made of a time-tested material that has never been shown to cause an allergic reaction. At last report, the company that makes SoftForm was in the process of developing a larger implant that can be used underneath the lip mucosa to provide lip augmentation.

AlloDerm

AlloDerm is a skin grafting material used for treating burn patients and for periodontal surgery, as well as for cosmetic and reconstructive surgery. It is made from human donor skin from which the epidermis and all of the cells in the dermis have been removed. What is left is the skin's protein framework. Once applied, the AlloDerm becomes part of the patient's own tissue.

Once processed, AlloDerm is freeze-dried and kept refrigerated until needed. It is then rehydrated in sterile saline solution to get a thin, pliable sheet that can be folded or rolled up like a jelly roll. It is then inserted under the skin via tiny incisions. Its uses in plastic surgery include lip augmentation, correcting depressed scarred areas (such as those left by acne), and nasal reconstruction.

Following the procedure, you are likely to have some swelling, which can be relieved by applying cold compresses. Your doctor will most likely give you a prescription for oral antibiotics to take for a few days along with antibiotic ointment to apply to the incision sites. A soft diet is recommended while healing. (See Fig. 4.5.)

COSMETIC TATTOOS

Like everyone else, our patients are way too busy these days. With demands from work, family, and just the general hassles of living, the extra minutes needed to keep looking good can be enough to push us over the edge. Who has time to put on eyeliner and have it look great every single time? Lipstick and eyebrow pencil can be a pain, and halfway through the day most of it has worn off, anyway.

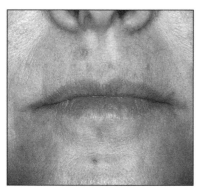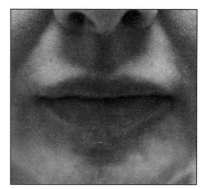

Figure 4.5 Forty-three-year-old female with AlloDerm augmentation (before and after).

Welcome to the age of the cosmetic tattoo. Since first learning that it existed back in 1988, I have met more and more patients who have had cosmetic tattooing such as permanent eyeliner and lip liner. It's so popular, in fact, that we have added it as an option during many procedures, including face-lifts. Our tattoo artist comes into the operating room after the surgery is complete and does the tattoo while the patient is still comfortably sedated or anesthetized. The pigment lasts usually between two and five years, with a touch-up procedure needed occasionally.

CHAPTER FIVE

Augmenting a Face-Lift

W HEN YOU CARE ABOUT HOW YOU LOOK (and who doesn't?), getting older can feel like being under siege. Gravity, a decrease in collagen and elastin, sun exposure, and our facial expressions gradually wear away that youthful glow and drag down our features until we begin to hate what we see in the mirror. But as countless satisfied patients can attest, you don't have to surrender without a fight. After all, you have modern technology and the cumulative experience of generations of plastic surgeons at your disposal.

We've already looked at one of the most powerful age-defying weapons, the face-lift. The main function of a face-lift is to tighten droopy skin on the face and neck. But there is more to aging than droopy skin, and a face-lift may not be enough to restore that youthful fullness and contour. Luckily, plastic surgeons have a range of techniques that they can use to help you reset aging's clock. Most can be performed either as stand-alone operations or in conjunction with the face-lift techniques discussed in chapter 4.

Like face-lifts, the procedures covered in this chapter are designed to rejuvenate the lower part of the face and the neck. Chapter 6 will discuss procedures for rejuvenating the upper portion of the face and the eyes.

LIPOSUCTION

Liposuction hails from France, where it was introduced in the early 1980s. Initially liposuction was used to reduce fat deposits on the torso and legs only. After extensive use over many years, we now feel confident and comfortable using it in the facial area.

To perform liposuction the surgeon makes a small incision in the area to be contoured and inserts a cannula that is attached to a suction machine or syringe. The cannula is passed back and forth under the skin to suction out the excess fat and "sculpt" the desired contours. Liposuction is usually performed under general anesthesia.

People who are good candidates for liposuction of the face and/or neck are those who have obvious fat deposits underneath the skin. For example, if you have fullness under your chin, you should be able to pinch the fat and actually feel it under the skin. If the problem is mostly fat, liposuction—rather than a face-lift—may be all that is needed to correct it.

Liposuction is not as good an option for people with a lot of excess skin. Some surgeons are using a similar technique, however, for patients who have excess skin but a minimal amount of fat. It involves passing a liposuction cannula just underneath the skin to scratch or irritate the undersurface. As the irritation heals it forms scar tissue that causes the skin to adhere to the underlying muscle tissue, which creates a lifting effect. A number of surgeons have reported excellent improvement in the appearance of the soft tissue of the neck region using this technique. (See Fig. 5.1.)

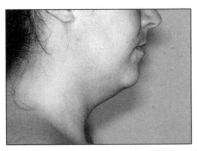 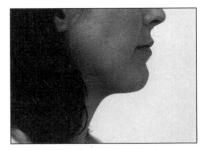

Figure 5.1 Thirty-five-year-old female with liposuction of neck only (before and after).

NECK CONTOURING AND TIGHTENING

I can't tell you how many times I have heard people plead with me to do something about their necks. This is the single most bothersome area for both men and women. For many people the problem is excess fat under the jawline, which creates what we call an "obtuse neck." There is very little definition along the jawline, and the person's face just seems to sort of flow down to the neck area. Sometimes the problem is not excess fat but droopy skin that hangs down under the jaw—the dreaded "turkey neck." Many people also complain about wrinkles around the neck, which I call "necklace wrinkles."

Most of the patients I see for neck problems range from their early forties to mid- seventies, but some are as young as their mid-twenties. They are not necessarily people who are aging ahead of their time or are seriously overweight. Instead, they have a genetic predisposition for developing an obtuse neck. (See Fig. 5.2.)

Neck and jaw problems can be addressed by liposuction alone (this usually works only in younger patients), by a neck and/or face-lift, or a combination of the two. In some cases, adding a chin implant will improve the results even further. These procedures are frequently combined with a face-lift operation. Some patients with significant neck deformities and skin aging may require secondary

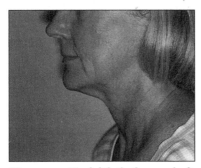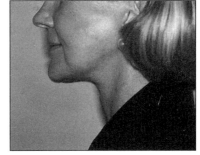

Figure 5.2 Neck lift (before and after).

face-lifting techniques where skin is actually re-excised at the area underneath the neck region.

THE Z-PLASTY

A simple alternative to a full face-lift operation is direct excision of neck skin using a method called Z-plasty. This is because of the zigzag incision used in the procedure. It is used because the scar from a straight-line incision would slowly contract, thus pulling the chin down toward the chest wall—not something to look forward to! The multiple Zs in the zigzag incision disperse the scar tissue formation and prevent this contraction effect.

Z-plasty can provide a nice improvement—in some cases even better than what could be achieved with the full face-lift technique. I usually reserve this approach for men in their fifties, sixties, and seventies. Most men are very happy with the final result. It is especially nice for older patients who may not be healthy enough for a full face-lift, such as men with high blood pressure.

Z-plasty can also be used as a secondary procedure on patients who have had previous face-lifts. It provides a way to improve the neck area without having to pull up on the cheek skin again, which would create in an unnatural, stretched appearance. For example, a woman once came to see me who had undergone a face-lift and some laser resurfacing about a year earlier. She had waited a long time to have these procedures done, so the aging effects were pretty significant by the time of surgery. Six months after her face-lift she looked fabulous. However, by one year post-op she had just a little bit of excess skin under her neck, which really bothered her. So we just excised it, worked with the muscles some more, and she had a beautiful—and natural-looking—result.

CHEEK LIFTS

Much as we might hate to think about fat serving any useful purpose, it is part of what gives our faces their definition and contour. This is particularly true in the cheek area. In young people, the fatty layer is attached high on the face, giving the cheeks a healthy fullness. As we get older those attachments loosen, the cheek starts to droop, and the nasolabial creases get deeper. If you're past your late thirties, take a look in any mirror, even your favorite, and you will see what I'm talking about. The droop in your cheeks makes you look tired and older. Use your hands to push your cheeks up toward your eyes, and see how much happier your face looks.

Several techniques can be used to help regain some of that youthful fullness without having to prop your cheeks up with your hands. One solution is cheek implants, which are described below under Facial Implants. Two other approaches are mid-cheek lifts and internal cheek lifts.

Mid-Cheek Lift

For this procedure, an incision is made beneath the lower eyelashes. The tissue of the cheek is lifted off the bony tissue and repositioned, and any excess skin is removed. If there is quite a bit of excess skin it may be necessary to do a lift in the temporal area as well. Combining a mid-cheek lift with a temporal lift gives an absolutely beautiful result to this area of the cheek along with the temporal and eye region. This is also called a subperiosteal face-lift, or cheek suspension. Temporal lifts are discussed in chapter 6. (See Fig. 5.3.)

Mid-cheek lifts can be performed separately or in combination with a face-lift or other procedures. The mid-cheek lift has almost revolu-

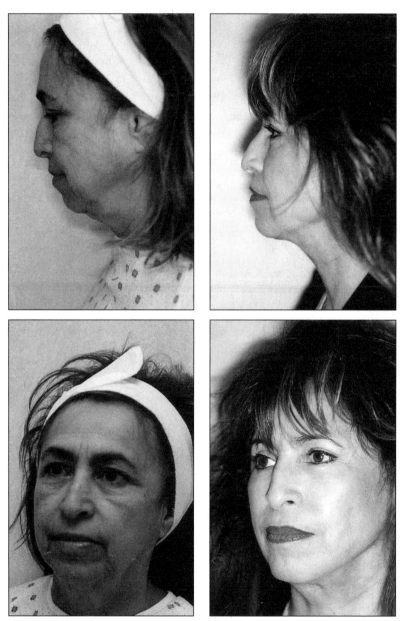

Figure 5.3 Before and after mid-cheek lift with upper and lower lid blepharoplasty.

tionized the overall face-lift by improving the eye and lip regions and the nasolabial fold along with the cheek area. The hollowness that was common with lower lid blepharoplasty can be eliminated with this lift.

Internal Cheek Lift

Internal cheek lifts are performed during a face-lift, after the incision has been made. In this procedure, the surgeon uses the incision under the eye to lift the cheek tissue and suture it to the undersurface of the face-lift flap; it is suspended when the skin is lifted and draped back. A variation on this theme is imbrication, in which the surgeon rolls the cheek tissue up and sews it in a horizontal roll to give fullness to the cheek tissue (similar to a cheek implant).

Getting Rid of That "Wind Tunnel" Effect

Cheek lifts can also counteract the flattening effect of a standard face-lift, thus avoiding the "wind tunnel" look. The reason for this is simple. In a face-lift, the skin and underlying tissue are pulled back toward the ear. But as we age, our skin droops down toward our feet, not away from our ears. A cheek lift takes this into consideration, lifting up tissue that has dragged down. Take a minute to look in a mirror and with your finger press on your cheek and elevate your cheek toward your eye. See what I mean?

I often have patients show up ten years after having had a face-lift, saying that they need another one. Most of the time, though, what they really need is a cheek lift. A perfect example of this is a woman who came to see me about six months ago. She was in her late sixties and had had a face-lift done three years earlier by a prominent local surgeon. She looked good, but something was missing. There were big hollows under her eyes and her cheeks still drooped. Even worse, she had a "plastic surgery look" that was obvious from across the room. It took me a while to persuade her that what she needed was a mid-cheek lift, but she finally decided to go through with it. Talk about transformation! Four months after having the procedure, this woman could be a poster child for mid-cheek lifts. She looks fantastic—not just younger, but healthy, vibrant, beautiful, and completely natural. Needless to say, she is thrilled with her appearance.

Be forewarned, however, that the recovery period for a cheek lift is fairly long. Although some fullness will be apparent pretty quickly, it will be a good three to four months before the final results can be appreciated. For the first couple of months, you may wonder whether it was worth it and if you will ever look any better. But believe me, you will, and you'll be glad you signed up for it and stuck it out.

FACIAL IMPLANTS

You've seen facial implants many times before, though probably without realizing it. Not to name names, but not all of those high cheekbones and wonderful facial contours that we see on magazine covers and fashion show runways are due to great genes. At least some of them have been augmented with implants. It isn't just fashion models and movie stars who can benefit from implants, however. Implants can also recreate the fullness and definition a face had in its youth but that has been eroded by age.

Cheek Implants

High, full cheeks give the face a healthy, youthful appearance. Sometimes a cheek lift is not enough to bring back that youthful look. In those cases cheek implants are a great option. I've had patients show up in my office two years after having face-lifts by other surgeons, wanting to know how they can look younger. Many times, small implants in the proper spots are all that is needed.

A cheek implant helps give fullness to the cheek area. It is especially great for patients with long, thin, drawn faces. They almost look haggard or sickly in appearance. Adding fullness to this area makes the face look more youthful and much healthier in appearance overall.

This was certainly true of Frank, a nice-looking man in his late thirties who was very concerned about the dark circles underneath his eyes and who came to me wanting to "have his eyes done." After evaluating him, I determined that it wasn't really the dark circles that were the problem. It was the loss of fullness in his cheek region that was causing him to look old, haggard, and tired. He didn't need either a face-lift or an "eye job." What he needed was fullness in his cheeks. By placing implants in his cheeks, we got rid of his nasolabial folds and de-emphasized the dark circles and puffiness under his eyes. As a result, he looked healthier and more energized—the way all of us want to look! Every one of my patients who received cheek implants has been very happy with them. (See Fig. 5.4.)

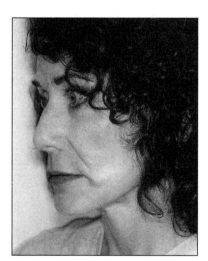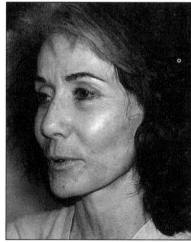

Figure 5.4 Sixty-three-year-old female with cheek implants in combination with a mini-lift (before and after). Overall, this rejuvenation of the face results in a much healthier appearance.

Cheek implants are usually inserted by making incisions in the mouth and placing them on top of the bony tissue of the cheek. If a face-lift is being performed at the same time, some surgeons will slip them through the face-lift incision. If this is done, however, the implants cannot be placed just underneath the skin and subcutaneous tissue. They need to sit right on top of the bony tissue, otherwise there is a significant risk that the implants will become displaced. Another approach is through an eyelid incision, which is often used if the implant surgery is being combined with a lower lid blepharoplasty. There is some risk of displacement with this incision as well.

When performed alone, cheek implant surgery is usually done under general anesthesia, although intravenous sedation is possible. I would not do it under straight local anesthesia. It is usually an outpatient procedure and takes about one to one and a half hours. You should be able to return to work about five days after surgery although your face will be quite swollen for two or three weeks. You will look as if you had your wisdom teeth removed, and an awkward smile is common but gets better over time. It may be two to three months before it looks fully natural.

During the early recuperation period, you will need to stay on antibiotics and use mouthwash frequently, especially right after eating. I usually have my patients stay on clear liquids for about a week after surgery. Most surgeons use dissolving sutures that will not need to be removed. Postsurgical infections are rare as long as the patient follows the antibiotic and mouthwash regimen faithfully. If an infection does occur, it presents itself as facial swelling around the cheek or eye area. Occasionally an infection is severe enough that the implant must be removed, but this is rare.

Chin Implants

Just as cheek implants can improve the mid-facial region, chin implants can help improve a patient's overall profile by improving its balance. A face is said to be in balance if you can draw an imaginary vertical line from the top of the forehead through the top of the nose, the upper lip, and the most prominent point of the chin. If a chin is set back or is too short or too long, it looks off-balance and destroys the overall facial symmetry. If you have what we call an obtuse-angle neck and a small chin, it may look as though the problem is entirely with your neck, when in fact it is a combination of a small chin and a neck problem.

A chin implant can improve the prominence of a small or setback chin, giving a better, more balanced look to the neck area and making the entire face-lift look better. Of course, the implant needs to be properly sized to your face and gender. A feminine face will tend to have a smaller chin, while a masculine chin will be stronger and more prominent. Some men go a step further, opting for the "chiseled manly look" seen on the covers of some men's magazines. The implants used to achieve this look are quite large, and are inserted through incisions made inside the mouth. A pocket is created on the outside of the jawline for the implant. This can make a soft jaw look much more masculine with definite angular contouring.

A chin implant takes anywhere from forty-five minutes to an hour to insert. The procedure can be done with local anesthetic, intravenous sedation, or general anesthesia. Recovery is pretty rapid, and most patients return to work within a week, although it is necessary to stay on a liquid diet for about ten days after surgery. With any type of facial implant it helps to be a ventriloquist since the less you move your facial muscles during the healing process, the better.

In addition to using implants, some surgeons perform craniomaxillofacial cosmetic surgery, in which the bones are repositioned in order to reshape the face and add desired fullness. The repositioned bones are held in place with plates and screws. This aggressive, involved, and time-consuming approach is not appropriate in most cases, but it can produce dramatic results when done properly.

Overall, my preference is for alloplastic (off-the-shelf) implants. They are predictable, easily inserted, and present fewer problems with resorption, which can occur with bony reconstruction.

Types of Facial Implants

Technological advances have improved facial implant options greatly over the last decade or so. The early implants were generally too small and not accurately shaped for the mid-facial region. Many of my patients with implants that are ten or more years old are having them redone because there are so many more anatomically appropriate shapes and sizes available.

Historically, a number of different materials have been used for implants, including ceramics, acrylic resins, ivory, and metal. Currently, the two types of alloplastic implants most commonly used in the United States are rubberized silicone and Proplast, a polymerized tetrafluorocarbon. Other implant materials include Gore-Tex and something called Porex, which is firmer and less resilient than the other types. Another type of implant, Supramed, is more commonly used in European countries.

Each surgeon will have his or her preferred type or types. Silicone and Proplast, for example, each offer different advantages and disadvantages. Silicone implants are preferred by most surgeons. They are nonporous and therefore more resistant to infection. They are also firmer and less fragile than Proplast implants, which makes them easier to place in the facial area. By contrast, Proplast is more porous, which allows tissue to grow into and around the implant. This helps the implant to stay in place, but it also creates a higher risk of infection. Further, the rapid tissue ingrowth can make the implant more difficult to remove if it does become infected.

JAW RECONTOURING

A person with an extremely prominent jaw is said to have mandibular hypertrophy or masseter muscle hypertrophy. Although some men feel that having a prominent jaw makes them look stronger and more masculine, others are bothered by it. This condition is common in the Asian population, and as a result, jaw recontouring is performed frequently in Asia, and especially in Korea. To perform the procedure, incisions are made inside the mouth, excess muscle and bone are removed, and the area is contoured. Most patients have an initial seven-day recovery period, followed by about a month of full recovery.

LIP AUGMENTATION

Lip augmentation is one of the most popular procedures in our practice (for which I have the models on the covers of fashion magazines to thank). As our mouth and lips age, we lose some of the fullness that makes them look young and "pouty." Take a look at some young people next time you're in the grocery store. Besides their skin, the thing that makes their faces seem most youthful is their lips. As we age, our lips shrink and vertical wrinkles form within the lip border. Lipstick starts to bleed, and our mouths just look more tired. This is why I often recommend that patients who are having any kind of face rejuvenating procedure think seriously about lip augmentation as well. I'm not talking huge, here, unless you really want it. But it's amazing what adding a little collagen or fat to your lips can do to make your whole face look more youthful. I think it's great that a relatively small procedure can impart such beautiful improvement to a face.

In chapter 4, we talked about various nonsurgical methods that can be used for lip augmentation. These include collagen, Dermalogen or Autologen injections, fat injections, and soft implants such as SoftForm or AlloDerm. If you have injectable implants, make sure that the doctor injects not just the lip border but also the lip muscle. This will bulk up the tissue and create a beautiful lip. I guarantee you'll like the results. (See Fig. 5.5.)

Regarding SoftForm implants for lip augmentation: The manufacturer originally recommended putting the implant right at the vermilion border of the lip, but this gave the lip an unnatural, accentuated appearance. In our practice, we place the SoftForm tubes

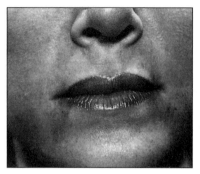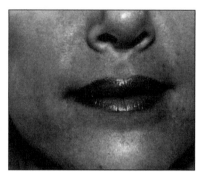

Figure 5.5 Lip augmentation with AlloDerm (before and after).

in the bulky tissue of the lip itself, which provides more natural results. The manufacturer has evidently realized the benefits to be derived from this placement because they are currently developing a
thicker tube that can be inserted in the bulk of the lip tissue to provide a pleasing fullness. In rare cases, SoftForm implants can become exposed. To correct this, the surgeon excises a portion of the
implant and recloses the opening in the lip. Even more rarely, a
patient's body will reject the material and the entire implant will
have to be removed.

In addition to collagen, fat, and soft implants, there are a couple
of surgical options that provide longer-lasting effects. These include
dermal fat grafts and lip lifts.

Dermal Fat Grafts

In this technique the surgeon removes fatty and dermal skin tissue
from one part of the face and places it surgically under the skin of
the lips to create fullness. This is a great technique to combine with
a face-lift because tissue removed during the face-lift operation can
be used to plump up the lips. Some surgeons use excess skin that
they have cut away from the face. Others "borrow" tissue from another area, such as the fascia, or covering, of the temporalis muscle
during the face-lift procedure.

This procedure takes approximately one hour. It can be done using either local anesthetic or general anesthesia.

Lip Lift

Probably the most involved procedure for lip augmentation is a lip lift. In this procedure, the surgeon outlines a new lip border above the existing one. (Make sure you get a chance to approve the outline before proceeding with the surgery. It should be precisely symmetrical.) The skin between the existing lip border (called the vermilion) and the new border is removed. Then the lip tissue is stretched and sutured into place. The sutures are left in place for seven days.

A similar technique is used to enlarge the lower lip. The surgeon excises a strip of skin from corner to corner of the mouth that is twice as wide as the desired size. The lip tissue is stretched to the new vermilion and sutured in place.

With either procedure, the lips will be swollen and sore for a week or longer. Cold compresses can help to reduce the initial swelling, and most people can return to work within a day or two. Most patients also experience a temporary loss of sensation at the incision site, but this usually resolves within a month or two. At the very least, there will be a visible line along the incision; some people will develop scar tissue in this area.

V-Y Plasty

Another technique used to create fullness in the upper lip is the V-Y plasty. In this procedure an incision is made in the upper lip to create V-shaped flaps, which are reoriented to create fullness. V-Y plasty is often performed as part of other lip augmentation procedures such as inserting SoftForm implants.

CHAPTER SIX

Procedures for the Upper Face

W E AGE ALL AT ONCE, not one body part at a time. So anyone who is contemplating having plastic surgery to look younger —and any surgeon who performs such surgery—must take into consideration the patient's entire appearance. The tendency, though, is for people to focus on the one or two features that bother them the most without realizing what else about their faces makes them look older.

In my experience, most people seem to be bothered by their necks more than anything else, and so they think that a face-lift and neck contouring will give them the look they want. But face-lifts and the other techniques we've discussed so far address only the lower two-thirds of your face. If your upper face is also showing the effects of aging, a face-lift alone can have the ironic effect of making the rest of your face look even older by comparison. Plus, your face will look oddly out of balance, as if you are two ages at once.

For this reason, many people opt to have a brow lift or forehead lift done at the same time as a face-lift. Conversely, some people may benefit more from having a brow lift and/or eyelid surgery *instead* of a face-lift. This is why it is so important to analyze your face as a whole—working with your surgeon—in order to decide which procedure or procedures will give you the results you want.

This chapter discusses procedures used to correct aging on the top part of the face and around the eyes: the brow lift or forehead lift, the temporal lift, and upper and lower blepharoplasty, or eyelid lifts.

THE IMPORTANCE OF EYEBROWS

Although most people probably don't realize it, our eyebrows have a major effect on our appearance — not just regarding how young or old we look but also what sort of mood or personality our face conveys. (See Figs. 6.1 and 6.2.) They can make us look happy or angry, sad or bewildered, rested or tired. Actors, artists, clowns, and cartoonists are quite aware of the eyebrows' importance for displaying emotion. They can convey everything from fear, to sadness, to joy, to surprise, just from changing the position of their eyebrows.

As we age, the region of the eyebrows typically begins to droop. If your brows droop to or below the orbital rim (the upper bony portion of the eyebrow rim), then your face can take on a stern, sinister, or unhappy appearance regardless of your current emotions — sadness, anger, excitement, or none of the above. Eyebrows that hang below the orbital rims of the skull are said to be "ptotic." *Ptotic* (pronounced "totic"; the *p* is silent) means prolapsed, or falling. Because we associate lowered brows with frowning, the effect of ptotic eyebrows is to make people appear chronically angry, brooding, or tired, regardless of how they actually feel.

One day after a Rotary Club luncheon meeting where I had spoken about plastic surgery, a man came up to me in the parking lot. Without stopping to introduce himself, he blurted, "I look so angry and sinister, Doctor, and I'm not like that! Can you make me look happier?" This man had very droopy eyebrows that loomed over his eyes like hoods. He did indeed look angry but was in fact a very jovial person whose face didn't fit his personality in any way. He was the perfect candidate for a brow lift. Needless to say, he made an appointment, the operation was performed, and he was delighted with his new look. His whole face had a softer appearance — not feminine, just natural and calm.

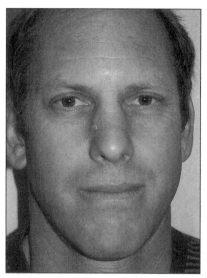

Figure 6.1 Forty-eight-year-old male with a T- shaped brow consistent with the aesthetically pleasing male brow.

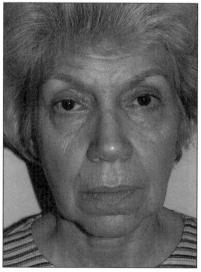

Figure 6.2 Sixty-eight-year-old female with a Y-shaped brow consistent with the aesthetically pleasing female brow.

IDENTIFYING THE PROBLEM

During the first consultation with a plastic surgeon, patients frequently focus just on their problem brow and excess skin around their eyes. They ask to just have their eyes done. It's important for you and your surgeon to determine whether in fact it is just your eyes or your forehead that is the problem. The best way to do this is to pull your brows up to their proper position and see if this eliminates the excess skin on the eyelid. If it does, then a brow lift is all you need. If some excess skin remains, then you will probably want to have a combination procedure that includes both a brow lift and a blepharoplasty (eyelid lift).

Take a look in the mirror and see where your brows line up. Are they hanging down over your eyes? Is one eyebrow higher than the other? (This can also be an indicator that a brow lift is in order.) If you have extremely deep forehead creases, you likely have droopy eyebrows as well and would most likely be a good candidate for a brow lift.

A word of caution: Most people, when they are looking in the mirror or having a picture taken, unconsciously raise their eyebrows, so a diagnosis of brow ptosis is not really valid unless the patient is holding quite still. During consultations I usually massage patients' foreheads with my fingers and then let them take a peek in the mirror to see the true position of their eyebrows.

THE BROW LIFT OR FOREHEAD LIFT

The brow lift is designed specifically to treat the tired, stern, angry look of the upper face. In addition to reducing or eliminating hooding, droopy eyebrows, it also reduces forehead creases and frown lines caused by overactive muscles (a condition called hypertrophy). The result is a face that looks more alert, serene, and youthful.

Brow lifts have been around for some time, but they have become more and more popular over the past ten years. Famous plastic surgeons such as Sam Hamra and Peter McKinney have realized that a face-lift alone does not completely rejuvenate the face, while combining the two operations can significantly improve a patient's overall appearance.

Candidates for brow lifts range from age thirty-eight or so and higher. Younger patients can often benefit from the minimally invasive endoscopic approach, where minimal incisions are used to elevate the brow, or a temporal lift. Older patients will require more involved techniques, generally with a larger incision at or above the hairline.

When patients come to see me about their eyebrows or forehead, I spend a fair amount of time evaluating what part of the brow actually needs to be lifted, and how far. Some patients say, "Dr. Henry, just lift them a little bit." Others want them raised significantly. Each case is unique, and it is critical to let your doctor know your feelings about the anticipated outcome. I usually position patients in front of a mirror and elevate the skin with my hands, to show them what they may look like with a brow lift or a temporal lift. It's important not to lift the brows too high, especially the inner brow, as this can make a person look permanently surprised, worried, bewildered, or uncertain. A well-trained plastic surgeon knows exactly where they should be positioned. (See Fig. 6.3.)

If a brow lift is being done in combination with an upper eyelid lift, the brow lift should be done first. This avoids the possibility of overcorrection, which can leave a patient looking permanently surprised or even unable to close her eyes.

Another issue in a brow lift is symmetry, or the lack of it. Most people's eyebrows are at least somewhat asymmetrical prior to surgery, and they may be asymmetrical after surgery as well. If you decide to have this operation, be sure to talk to your surgeon ahead of time about any asymmetry between your eyebrows and your expectations regarding this.

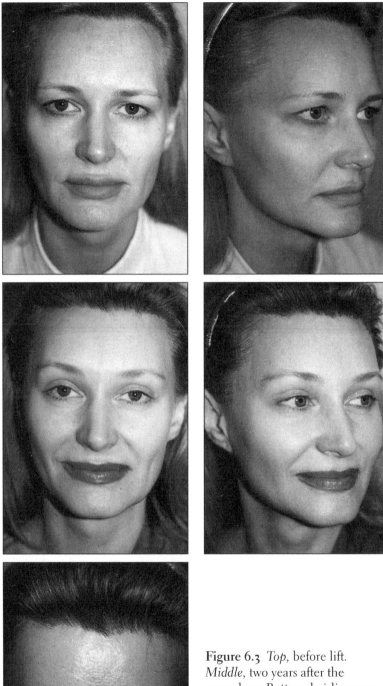

Figure 6.3 *Top*, before lift.
Middle, two years after the
procedure. *Bottom*, hairline scar,
two years after the procedure.

Muscle Removal or Resectioning

Inappropriate expressions can occur after a brow lift, which is why your surgeon needs to work closely with you to determine the most appropriate incision and procedures to use. You want your face to look natural and not permanently surprised, startled, sad, or bewildered. One important decision is whether to remove or weaken the corrugator and/or the frontalis muscles.

The Corrugator Muscles   These tiny muscles sit between your eyebrows and are responsible for the creases that appear between your eyebrows, when you frown. Removing or weakening them lessens or eliminates the face's ability to form the creases—a result that many women, at least, find desirable. On the other hand, many men, and some women, do not want to lose any facial expressiveness.

The Frontalis Muscle   The frontalis is the main large muscle of the forehead. This is the muscle you use to raise your eyebrows, which is also the action that eventually creates lines across your forehead. One way to soften or eliminate the lines is to inhibit the muscle's function. This can be done temporarily using Botox injections, or permanently, by transecting (cutting across) the muscle in one or more places. Surgeons tend to do this more aggressively in women because women, in general, prefer to reduce their forehead creases as much as possible. Men, on the other hand, tend to not mind some creasing. The frontalis muscle is never completely removed because doing so would create an unnatural absence of expression.

Locating the Brow Lift Incision   Several different incision locations can be used for brow lifts. The one your surgeon uses will depend on a range of factors such as the number and depth of your wrinkles, your complexion type, and the location of your hairline.

The bicoronal method is the one most commonly used today. It consists of a single incision extending from ear to ear, about 5 to 7 centimeters behind the hairline. The greatest advantage to the bicoronal incision is that it is hidden in the hairline. If your forehead is rather broad and long, your surgeon may elect to use an incision that begins right at the hairline, called a pretrichlear incision. The incision can also be placed along the hairline, right behind it, or using some combination of these two.

Another option is the direct brow incision. In this technique, incisions are made just above each eyebrow and excess skin is excised to help reposition the eyebrow. Although this might seem the most direct way to elevate the brow, it does not allow removal of the corrugator muscles. Yet another possibility is placing the incision inside an already existing forehead crease. This is a good approach for a man who is balding or whose hairline is receding. Endoscopic incisions are another possibility for people who don't have enough hair to cover a large incision (see below).

The Procedure

Once the incision is made, the skin is elevated above the skull and smoothed back toward the top of the head to lift the brows, much the same way the skin is smoothed in a face-lift. If the patient and surgeon decide it is appropriate, the corrugator muscles are removed or dissected at this point. The surgeon may also weaken the frontalis muscle during this stage. Then the skin flap is redraped into position, the excess skin excised, and the incision closed. Most surgeons close the incision in layers. For the deeper layers they use a subcuticular stitch, which will be absorbed by the body as it heals. The outer layers are closed with either staples or sutures. Staples are generally preferred because if the tissue swells, the staples will also swell. This helps prevent injury to fine hair follicles on the scalp, thus preventing hair loss along the incision. Staples usually remain in place for about eight to ten days.

The surgeon may or may not use a dressing on the incision. I usually dress patients in a "mummy wrap" in the operating room.

They go home wearing the same bandage and return the following morning for me to remove it. One or more tubes may also be inserted to drain off fluid accumulation. If used, these are removed during either first or second day post-op.

A brow lift operation takes anywhere from an hour and a half to three hours and can be performed under either general anesthesia or intravenous sedation with local anesthetic. Most patients go home about an hour and a half after surgery. Post-op, you will be a little black and blue around your eyes and will have some swelling in that area. Ice compresses will help decrease the bruising and swelling. As with a face-lift, you will need to sleep with your head elevated for a week or so following surgery to keep down swelling and prevent complications due to bleeding. We tell our patients they can wash their hair the day after surgery and wear it the way they normally do.

Most patients experience some eye dryness following a brow lift. This can be helped with eye drops such as artificial tears. Patients who had dry-eye problems prior to surgery may find that it gets worse, so be sure to tell your surgeon ahead of time if this may be a problem for you.

Following a brow lift, many patients find that the skin in front of the scalp incision is slightly numb. In most cases, the nerves rejuvenate and numbness decreases over time, though it can be permanent. You'll need to be careful with curling irons and hair dryers during the healing phase. Occasionally, there can be temporary hair loss near the incisions, but this usually improves over the next four to six months. The risk of hair loss is greater in smokers—another reason smoking and plastic surgery don't mix! Some surgeons place micro–hair tufts along the incision—a new technique that helps eliminate any possible hair loss. Using Rogaine or Propecia before and after surgery may also help.

The recovery period for a brow lift is comparable to a face-lift: three to five days for initial recovery, and complete recovery in ten to twelve days. Most patients return to work within one to two weeks. Patients look better right away. Forehead creases are eliminated for some patients and significantly reduced for others. Most importantly, the tired, angry look is replaced by a serene, more youthful one. Most patients are very happy after a brow lift. In fact, I have had many patients tell me that they are glad that I recommended it to them as they had never understood why they looked angry, sad, or tired. I remember one patient who, after her brow lift, said that when she got mad at her kids, they just laughed at her because she looked so pleasant and cheerful—even when she was angry!

Occasionally brow droopiness may recur, thus requiring a second operation, but this is rare. Usually once a brow lift has been done, it lasts a lifetime.

Endoscopic Brow Lift

Have you ever heard of removing a gallbladder via a small incision? To do this, a camera is attached to a long narrow tube called an endoscope. When the endoscope is inserted through a tiny incision, it enables a surgeon to see and work inside the abdomen. One or more other small incisions are used to insert the special instruments needed to perform the procedure. This micro-approach is being used in more and more types of surgery and plastic surgery is no exception. Though some surgeons are using endoscopes for other procedures, including face-lifts, they have become almost routine for treating brow ptosis, corrugator muscle hypertrophy (frown lines), and frontalis muscle hypertrophy (forehead creases).

For this technique, the surgeon makes about five small incisions in the area where a brow lift incision would normally be located. The skin is then lifted off the bony tissue, pulled up, and tacked down to the deeper tissue of the forehead. There are now new fixation devices that can be secured underneath the skin, but some surgeons prefer to use external devices that are removed after two or three weeks. The corrugator muscles (the muscles that create the frown lines between the eyebrows) may also be weakened or removed with special scissors.

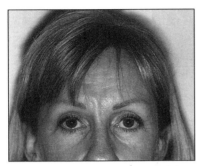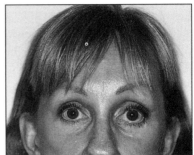

Figure 6.4 Endoscopic brow lift to correct frown lines between eyebrows (before and after).

An endoscopic brow lift can be performed under either general anesthesia or intravenous sedation and local anesthetic. The procedure can take anywhere from forty-five minutes to three hours depending upon the surgeon's ability. Postoperative bruising is usually minor and recovery tends to be faster than with traditional brow lifts. Endoscopic lifts tend to be slightly more expensive than a regular brow lift. (See Fig. 6.4.)

Many surgeons have adopted endoscopic brow lifts for patients who do not want the ear-to-ear incision of a traditional brow lift. However, not everyone is a good candidate for this technique. Endoscopic brow lifts are most effective in younger patients who do not require large corrections. People who have deep forehead creases, very high foreheads, or significant brow ptosis (droopiness) generally need to have the full incision.

Temporal Lift

Sometimes patients come to me saying, "Just pull up my eyebrow like this," and demonstrate by pulling the skin up with their fingers. If a full brow lift is not needed or desired, a more subtle effect can be achieved with a temporal lift. This is an especially good option for people in their mid-thirties to early forties whose brows are drooping sideways toward their temples. Lateral brow ptosis, as it is referred to, makes people look very tired and sad. In a temporal lift, the skin is drawn up from the eyebrow area, lifting the eyes to a higher level. With minimal elevation we can open up the eyes and brow area so that patients look not only younger but happier and more energetic.

A temporal lift is easy to perform and can be done under direct local anesthesia, intravenous sedation, or even general anesthesia. The procedure is similar to a brow lift, but the incisions are placed in the temporal area only. Usually an incision is made about three finger widths back of the hairline. The skin is lifted and the area undermined. Then the excess skin is removed and the incision closed with sutures and/or staples. The identical procedure is then performed on the opposite side.

The benefit of a temporal lift is that it avoids the ear-to-ear incision required for a brow lift while still providing distinct elevation in the area of concern. Most patients are extremely happy with this less invasive procedure, but you must be a candidate for it. Not all patients are good candidates. Some patients may really need a full brow lift. This is something that will need to be evaluated by your plastic surgeon.

The initial recovery period for a temporal lift is around four to five days. Bruising can range from minimal to significant. As with other forehead lifting procedures it is common for patients to develop temporary numbness around the incision.

Botox Injections: The Temporary Solution

Occasionally, patients decide against having a brow lift either because they are concerned about the incision or just not quite ready. I often recommend Botox injections to these patients so that they can develop an understanding of what a brow lift could do for their overactive forehead muscles. As you'll recall from chapter 4, Botox can be used to temporarily paralyze the corrugator and/or frontalis muscles, thus relaxing frown lines and forehead creases. This gives an effect that is similar to a surgical brow lift, but temporary. Unfortunately, Botox won't do anything for droopy eyebrows.

BLEPHAROPLASTY

Our eyes are our most important feature and the part of the face that other people look at first. Your eyes relay subtle messages about how you feel and what is going on. They tell others if you are happy, sad, or scared. The eyes also convey an overall sense of well-being or lack of it. Earlier we discussed the effects of eyebrow position in regard to your appearance. The next step is to make sure the eye region looks clean and unobstructed.

As I explained in chapter 2, the eyes are one of the first places to show the effects of aging, particularly the upper and lower lids. Droopy, sagging, crepe-like eyelids can make people look tired, sick, and depressed, even when they feel great. This effect is created by excess skin. I have had patients actually grab the skin and pull it up, saying, "See, Dr. Henry, this is the stuff that bothers me." Women will often say that they can't use eye shadow anymore.

This isn't just a cosmetic issue (no pun intended!). Some older people have so much excess skin on their upper lids that they have trouble seeing. Nor do you have to be all that old to have eyelid problems. Many younger people wish they could get rid of those pouchy bags or dark rings under their eyes. For these reasons blepharoplasties, or eyelid lifts, are the most common of all plastic surgeries, accounting for more than fifty thousand procedures a year in the United States alone.

For such a simple operation, blepharoplasty can produce amazing results. Many surgeons believe that eyelid surgery does more to help a person look alert, attentive, and fresher, not to mention younger, than any other plastic surgery procedure. Except in younger people looking to get rid of the bags under their eyes, most people achieve optimum results by having both their upper and

lower lids done at the same time. Either or both procedures can easily be done at the same time as a face-lift or brow lift.

Upper Lid Blepharoplasty

As we age, the skin on our upper eyelids thins and develops fine
wrinkles rather like crepe fabric or paper. At the same time the area
around the eyes becomes puffy because the thin skin is less able to
restrain the fatty tissue underneath it. This crepiness and fullness
worsens over time, but it can be helped by having an upper lid blepharoplasty performed. (See Fig. 6.5.)

To perform this procedure, the surgeon first takes careful mea-
surements to determine how much skin should be removed. A small
incision is made in the eyelid crease, as shown in the following di-
agram, using either a scalpel or laser, and the excess skin is excised.
The surgeon may also remove some or all of two small fat pads in
the upper lid. These deposits, called the medial and central fat pads,
can make the eye look puffy. If there is fullness or puffiness near
the outer portion of the eye, it may also be necessary to reposition the
lacrimal gland, a tear-producing gland in the outer corner of the eyelid. The incision is then closed using fine sutures, which are removed
four to five days after surgery.

Upper lid blepharoplasty can be performed using a straight local
anesthetic or under intravenous sedation or general anesthesia depending on the patient's anxiety level. Discomfort following the
surgery is minimal. When I had mine done about ten years ago, it
was under straight local anesthesia, with a shot of Demerol to make
me a bit more relaxed.

Lower Lid Blepharoplasty

A person with excess skin, excess wrinkled muscle, or puffiness underneath the lower eyelid may be a good candidate for a lower lid
blepharoplasty. In this procedure the surgeon makes a small inci-

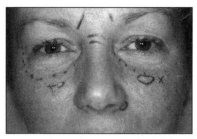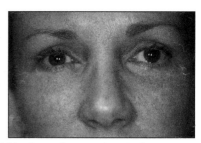

Figure 6.5 Before and after upper lid blepharoplasty and mid-cheek lower lid blepharoplasty. Notice improved youthfulness in lower lid using this technique. Older techniques produce a hollowness in the lower lid region that is more aging.

sion near the eyelid area, under the lash margin. The skin and the underlying muscle are lifted off to reveal any excess fat. We all have three small fat pads under each eye. The puffier the eyes, the larger the fat pads. In a traditional blepharoplasty, where a mid-cheek lift is not being performed, this excess fat is removed. Then the surgeon tacks the outer corner of the eye against the orbital rim and excises excess skin or muscle tissue of the lower lid.

Another option for this condition, which was discussed in chapter 5, is a mid-cheek lift. Many surgeons are now opting to do the mid-cheek lift rather than a lower lid blepharoplasty as the results are generally much more aesthetically appealing. In a mid-cheek lift, most or all of the excess fat around the lower lid is left in place. The entire skin and soft tissue of the lower cheek region is then elevated and secured near the temple. This helps improve the nasolabial folds (the lines around the mouth that become increasingly noticeable with age). It also helps provide fullness to the cheek area and, overall, gives a healthy-looking appearance to the middle portion of the face.

An upper lid blepharoplasty takes about an hour to complete. A lower lid blepharoplasty takes about an hour to an hour and a half. Although upper lid blepharoplasties are sometimes performed using only a local anesthetic, most lower lid and combination procedures are done under intravenous sedation.

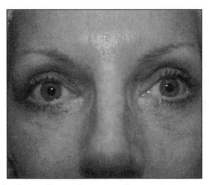

Figure 6.6 Lid blepharoplasty three weeks postsurgery.

Following surgery, the eyes will be swollen and black and blue. Cold compresses can help to alleviate the swelling and bruising. I have my patients dampen 4 × 4 gauze pieces and freeze them to make miniature ice compresses. Other surgeons use small balloons filled with frozen peas.

As with other facial surgery, patients need to sleep with their heads elevated for several nights following a blepharoplasty to keep down swelling and avoid complications due to bleeding. Most patients return to work in about a week. The eyes will remain puffy for a couple of weeks. (See Fig. 6.6.)

Another Approach—For Young Patients Only

Another operation I have used with some younger patients who do not have a lot of excess skin and rolls of excess muscle tissue is the transconjunctival approach, also called an incisionless blepharoplasty. In this operation the surgeon makes an incision on the inside of the eyelid and removes only the excess fat that is noticeable. No sutures are required.

The best candidates for this operation are people in their mid-twenties to early thirties whose problem is not excess skin as much as puffiness that may be either genetic or caused by allergies. When these patients hit their forties and fifties, they may need more extensive surgery in this area—either a mid-cheek lift or regular blepharoplasty.

OTHER PROCEDURES FOR THE UPPER FACE

Other procedures that are sometimes performed in conjunction with face-lift or brow lift surgery include a procedure to remove crow's-feet, forehead recontouring, and temporal fossa augmentation.

Removing Crow's-Feet

In our practice, many patients opt for Botox injections and/or laser resurfacing to help eliminate crow's-feet. There is a surgical procedure for this, however, called an orbicularis oculi myoplasty. The surgeon makes a cut across a portion of the eye muscle so that the fibers cannot connect. This decreases the function of the muscle somewhat, thus relaxing the surface wrinkles. This procedure is sometimes combined with a face-lift.

Forehead Recontouring

A major difference between the Neanderthals of thousands of years ago and modern *Homo sapiens* is that most members of our species do not have prominent foreheads that hang out over our eyes. Such a forehead can make a person look permanently angry, brooding, or even somewhat scary. This problem can be corrected with forehead recontouring. To achieve this, the surgeon makes an incision across the top of the forehead to expose the skull and then uses an instrument called a burr to shave down the brow bone.

Forehead recontouring may also be an option for a woman whose forehead gives her face a more masculine appearance than she would like. In the San Francisco area, where I live, we have a prominent surgeon whose practice consists largely of men who are in the process of being changed into women. His focus is on transforming masculine faces to feminine ones, which often includes recontouring their foreheads.

If you are interested in forehead recontouring, you will need to find someone who has experience with the procedure since it is not routinely performed by most plastic surgeons.

Temporal Fossa Augmentation

The *temporal fossa* is a region of the temple that, over time, starts to become indented. For most people, this doesn't happen until late old age, in their eighties or nineties. Some individuals, however, develop this indentation earlier, particularly people of Asian descent. The treatment recommended is to augment the indentations using either an implant or some other type of soft tissue that is inserted through an incision in the scalp.

CHAPTER SEVEN

Laser and Other Resurfacing Techniques

S O FAR WE HAVE LOOKED AT A VARIETY of procedures aimed at undoing the effects of gravity, overuse of facial muscles, and the loss of fat and collagen that happens as we age. But what about all those lip lines, fine wrinkles, age spots, and other problems that affect the skin's surface? Many of these flaws are not correctable with surgery. Instead, we need a way to remove those old, damaged skin layers and replace them with fresher, smoother, tighter skin.

Until a few years ago, plastic surgeons and dermatologists relied on phenol chemical peels or dermabrasion to improve surface wrinkles and remove age spots, acne scars, and other surface flaws. The biggest drawback as a result of these techniques was the potential for overlightening the skin, particularly in olive- and dark-complexioned patients. Since the mid-1990s, however, we have had another option: laser resurfacing. Laser treatments give a better result overall, with more uniform treatment of wrinkles and other skin imperfections. Although the possibility of overlightening still exists, it is significantly smaller compared to other methods.

Lasers have been used in medical applications since the sixties. But early lasers could not be used for cosmetic applications because they burned the skin. The carbon dioxide (CO_2) UltraPulse laser and the Erbium laser solve this problem by emitting high-energy beams in very short bursts. The energy bursts, in effect, vaporize the top layer of skin. But because they are so short their heat dissipates before harming the underlying tissue. At the same time, collagen bundles in the dermis are disrupted, which causes the skin to contract and tighten. After a healing period, the result is smoother, healthier, and younger-looking skin. Since this laser technology was introduced in the mid-1990s, thousands of patients have been treated safely with it.

WHAT CAN LASERS DO?

The CO_2 UltraPulse laser is the best thing going for getting rid of wrinkles including:

- Wrinkles around the mouth
- Crow's-feet
- Cheek wrinkles
- Most forehead wrinkles
- Wrinkles due to wrinkling your nose
- Wrinkles as a result of sun exposure

In some of our patients, laser resurfacing has actually improved upper eyelid skin redundancy, similar to what you receive from an upper lid blepharoplasty. Sometimes the skin-tightening effect of the laser lifts the eyebrows, providing an effect comparable to a formal brow lift. Sometimes the neck skin can tighten up as well, simulating a minilift. To achieve major changes in very droopy skin, however, laser resurfacing is probably not enough, and we have to consider more invasive procedures such as a face-lift.

Lasers can be used to improve or eliminate a whole assortment of other flaws such as age spots, freckles, pitted scars such as those from acne, tattoos, spider veins, redness caused by rosacea, and areas of hyper (too much) and hypo (too little) pigmentation.

The CO_2 Laser

The instrument we use for laser resurfacing is a CO_2 UltraPulse laser manufactured by the Coherent Medical Group. It consists of a box that produces a specific wavelength of light, which is emitted through a handheld device about the size and shape of a pencil. The "pencil" makes it easy for the surgeon to control the direction of the light beam with great precision and accuracy. The beam's intensity is controlled by a computer, which is operated by a technician under the doctor's direction.

The laser is easy to use and can be operated by anyone who has received training through a medical training course or a weekend course conducted by the manufacturer. Most of the physicians using CO_2 lasers are plastic surgeons, dermatologists, and ear, nose and throat surgeons who perform cosmetic surgery. They are also used by ophthalmologists and even some dentists. We often conduct evening or weekend seminars where we let patients see firsthand how a laser works. We call it our "tomato and eggplant show." With the help of our laser technician, we instruct patients on how to use the laser, and in a controlled setting allow them to do some "resurfacing" on vegetables.

As with any surgical procedure, however, it's important to make sure that your surgeon is qualified and experienced at operating the laser. We'll discuss this later when we talk about choosing a plastic surgeon in chapter 10. (See Figs. 7.1 and 7.2.)

The Erbium Laser

The Erbium laser is the latest thing on the antiwrinkle scene, having been introduced in 1997. Its benefits are supposed to be that it doesn't go as deep as the CO_2, meaning that there is less discomfort, less downtime for healing, and less redness—perfect for those who want results now and only have a few hours to recuperate from the procedure.

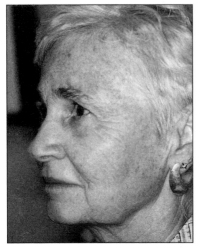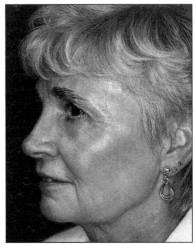

Figure 7.1 Before and after face-lifting techniques using full-face laser CO_2.

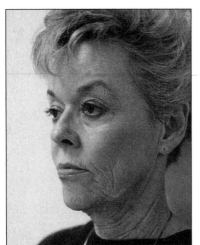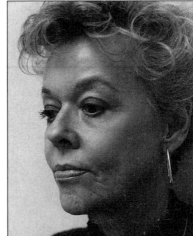

Figure 7.2 Before and after full-face laser CO_2. This sixty-three-year-old female wanted to get rid of her "wrinkles" but didn't want a face-lift. Postoperatively, she said she had been on a "vacation."

About two years ago, I was asked by one of the local laser companies to sponsor a course for the erbium laser. A doctor from Hollywood was coming to give us a hands-on demonstration, and I was definitely excited at the prospect. We had about thirty doctors and nurses scheduled to be with us on the big day. Heidi, one of our skin care specialists, signed up to receive a full-face Erbium resurfacing as part of the demonstration. She was forty-one at the time, and though she looked young for her age, she wanted to get rid of some wrinkles and freshen up her skin. The fancy doctor in charge of the seminar did her entire face under straight local anesthetic. Not only did she wiggle, but she was in extreme discomfort throughout the experience. Afterward she went through an entire week of healing, just as she would have with the CO_2 laser. And the final result? She was not as red as she would have been with a CO_2 laser treatment, but she also still had her wrinkles. In fact, except for the redness, you couldn't tell anything had been done.

So if you have significant wrinkles, consider the CO_2. There are recent changes being made to the Erbium that may make it better in the future. But just because the healing time is faster does not mean you will end up with the results that you expect. The persistence of redness is actually a good sign, and fortunately, it can be covered with makeup until it fades.

WHEN SHOULD LASER RESURFACING BE DONE?

There is no perfect age for having laser resurfacing done. Generally, our laser patients range from their late thirties to their eighties; the youngest to date has been a woman in her early thirties. Older patients are usually interested in dramatic improvement, which often means having a lifting procedure to tighten some of their excess skin prior to the laser work. Younger patients, on the other hand, are just beginning to see the effects of aging and want to intervene before those become too pronounced. These patients have more superficial wrinkling, which can be eliminated with some of the lighter laser techniques.

Thus, when a patient comes to my office saying, "I want to get rid of my wrinkles," I do an initial screening to determine what approach we should take. Would this person benefit from a surgical procedure that stretches out the skin, like a face-lift? Or is there wrinkling in areas that a lift won't correct? How does she feel about surgery? Some patients are open to the idea while others say flat out, "Forget it, I don't want a face-lift. I just want to get rid of the wrinkles on my cheeks and around my eyes and lips." It was for these patients that laser techniques were invented. But laser treatment can also greatly enhance the results of a face-lift. Laser resurfacing on top of a face-lift creates a refreshed appearance—the airbrushed look, only for real.

In our practice, we provide laser treatments both alone and in combination with a face-lift.

Full-Face Versus Partial Resurfacing

With chemical peels and dermabrasion, plastic surgeons and dermatologists often zeroed in on a particular area of the face. The most common place for resurfacing was the upper lip, where most of us develop fine lines as a result of smoking, muscle functioning, and aging.

When we first began performing laser treatments, we used the same approach, doing only certain areas of the face such as the area around the eyes or the lipstick "bleed" area. Or we would focus on specific lines, expecting them to go away. Now, however, the trend is to perform full-face resurfacing on the majority of patients. This is because experience has shown that patients who have only partial lasering end up with areas of demarcation—their faces have obvious boundaries between the lasered and unlasered portions. I remember one patient who wanted laser resurfacing around her mouth and forehead where she had a lot of wrinkles. She would not allow us to do a full-face laser, even though we tried to tell her it was what she needed. Well, of course, she healed with areas of demarcation and wound up having a second procedure over her whole face so that her skin would have a uniform appearance.

Combining Laser Resurfacing with a Face-Lift or Brow Lift

As we've seen, face-lift or brow lift surgery may not eliminate fine surface wrinkles or other flaws. For this reason, many people opt to have both a face-lift and resurfacing, using either the laser or a chemical peel. The result is a smoother, refreshed appearance. In our practice, I sometimes combine lasering the middle portion of the face with a brow lift or upper face-lift.

Resurfacing can be done at the same time as the face-lift, or as a separate procedure six to twelve weeks after the initial procedure. If both procedures are done at the same time, however, the surgeon needs to take special precautions since the skin is being hit with a double whammy. Its underside is being lifted off of the facial tissue, and the surface is being hit with laser energy. The result can be very upset skin and subsequent poor healing.

The solution is to vary the intensity of the laser energy used on different areas of the face depending on what other procedures have been performed and the thickness of the skin in each area. Generally, the full laser setting can be used on the nose, upper lip, and chin. The cheeks and neck require a much lower laser setting.

Lasers and the Neck

For patients who have a significant number of neck wrinkles, the laser can be extended down onto the area of the neck after administering to the face. As with facial laser resurfacing, neck lasering can help achieve an overall tightening of the neck skin. At this point in time, however, the procedure is controversial. The skin on our necks is more fragile than the skin on our faces, and it can be damaged easily by aggressive or overly zealous treatments, leading to poor wound healing and potentially serious scarring. Some surgeons will not even laser the neck region after a face-lift due to concerns regarding the healing process.

We happen to do neck lasering in our practice, but we are very cautious and conservative in our approach. We use it only following a face-lift in order to treat wrinkles not improved by surgery, and always follow exact parameters based on the initial studies that included neck lasering with facial resurfacing. The laser energy is decreased to about half the facial setting, and the laser energy is angled in a little different direction. We have had beautiful results using this conservative approach, with no complications during the healing period.

If you decide that this is a procedure you would like done, make sure your surgeon has experience doing it and that he or she will be extremely cautious with the settings.

A Note About Laser Resurfacing and Skin Cancer

Not long ago, the vice president of a prominent business in our community came to my office. He was in his late sixties and very concerned about the texture of his skin, which was severely damaged as a result of many years of sun exposure. He had had skin cancers removed from his face in the past and now had another one on his forehead that had recently been biopsied and determined to be positive.

The cancerous spot was excised, and six weeks later we did a full laser resurfacing of his face. Eight days later, the texture of his skin had improved tremendously. Not only had we improved his skin texture, but we had eliminated most, if not all, of the potentially cancerous growths on his face.

It's important to realize that laser resurfacing is not a cure-all for skin cancers—especially melanoma. If you have a raised patch of skin that appears irritated, you need to have it checked by a dermatologist. If it is malignant or potentially malignant, it will need to be removed. However, laser resurfacing may decrease the recurrence patterns of some superficial basal cell and squamous cell skin cancers. Ask your dermatologist or plastic surgeon about this.

THE PROCEDURE

Prior to laser resurfacing, most surgeons have patients prepare their skin by using Retin A or an alpha-hydroxy acid product for at least four to six weeks. (Since most of my patients have already been on glycolic acid or lactic acid for some time, they usually do not need to wait the extra four weeks.)

A few days before the procedure, we also start our patients on an antiviral medication such as Famvir or acyclovir, which they continue taking for a few days after surgery. This is to prevent herpes infections and is especially important for patients who have a history of cold sores or herpes infections inside or around their mouths. A herpes infection, if it occurs, usually sets in a few days after the laser procedure. It usually shows up as small ulcers on the lips, which then extend to other areas of the face. During the healing period, it's important to report *any and all* changes on your face to your doctor so that any infections can be treated immediately.

Local anesthetic is generally sufficient for lasering small areas, such as lip lines. A full-face laser takes approximately an hour and fifteen minutes and can be done under either intravenous sedation or general anesthesia. I do the majority of my laser resurfacing procedures under general anesthesia because I want my patients to have a comfortable experience. I have heard about some dermatologists who perform full-face lasering using only a local anesthetic and take up to three hours to complete the procedure. I don't recommend putting anyone through that experience. Three hours is an awfully long time to be wriggling on an operating room table.

Most laser procedures are pretty straightforward for me to perform, but perhaps that is because I've done so many of them. It's not a difficult operation, but it can lead to complications if not done properly, primarily infection and scarring. Because the laser's heat cauterizes the blood vessels in the skin, bleeding is not a problem, even in patients who are taking blood thinners, such as Coumadin.

Currently, two types of dressings are used for laser resurfacing patients: open and closed. In the open technique, as soon as the surgeon has completed the treatment, a special ointment is applied to the skin. This is repeated several times throughout the day. In between applications most surgeons have patients wash their skin with a mild cleanser.

In the closed technique, a dressing is cut specially to fit over the whole face. This dressing is laid over the face after surgery to block out air and collect the fluids that ooze from the skin. Some surgeons think that patients have less pain and discomfort with the closed technique. It carries a significantly higher risk of infection, however, so patients need to be watched carefully when using it. Also, the dressings tend to fall off in a couple of days anyway.

We use the open method with our patients, applying an antibiotic ointment such as Neosporin or bacitracin ointment immediately after the procedure. (For the occasional patient who exhibits a sensitivity to antibiotic ointments, we use petroleum jelly instead.) We also apply a copper-based cream that helps to speed healing and decreases the discomfort.

The procedure is conducted on an outpatient basis, and most patients go home directly afterward.

THE RECOVERY PERIOD

Recovery following laser resurfacing is pretty straightforward, but it can be rather upsetting to look at and pretty uncomfortable, especially for the first few days. Expect to lay low for at least a week after the procedure. Do not go outside. Do not go to the grocery store. Do not make appointments to see your friends. Expect to feel tired and worn out in addition to feeling as if you have the worst sunburn of your life. Your skin will feel tight, wet, and on fire. Most patients take some kind of painkiller for the first couple of days. I recommend keeping a big bowl of ice water right next to the bed along with a washcloth that you can dip into it and drape over your face. This, along with the copper cream, helps alleviate any discomfort quite a bit.

Most patients hate the way they look for the first two or three days following the procedure when their skin is swollen, weepy, and crusty. I get a lot of calls around the third day from patients saying, "I can't believe people do this and survive!" But by the sixth or seventh day, when things have started to turn the corner, they say they wished they'd done it sooner. By then the old skin has begun to peel, revealing brand new pink skin that glistens and is as smooth as glass.

It's important to avoid the sun for at least two or three months following any kind of skin resurfacing. If you must go outside during the day, wear sunglasses and a hat, and stay in the shade as much as possible. Sun exposure can cause hyperpigmentation (a darkening of the skin). For this reason, summer is the worst time to have laser work done. (I'm speaking from experience here. I had my laser work performed during the summer, and in California the sun can be pretty intense.) If you do end up with pigmentation problems such as demarcation lines, you can cause them to fade by applying a topical bleaching cream. This takes quite some time, however, so it's best to prevent the problems from happening in the first place.

Everyone has some redness following laser resurfacing, but it will improve with time. The average is two to three months, but some patients lose the redness within a month, and others have it for as long as six months. In my case, the pinkness lasted about sixteen weeks. I have never seen the redness persist indefinitely. A special mineral-based camouflage makeup is available that helps to lessen the redness. It can usually be worn by the seventh or eighth day.

MY EXPERIENCE WITH LASER RESURFACING

When I was growing up, especially during the sixth, seventh, and eighth grades, I longed for beautiful skin. Unfortunately, I was blessed with my father's genes, which meant that I was cursed with pimples. Naturally, I hated them like nobody's business and tried everything I could think of to get rid of them. Once I even sat under a sunlamp for a full hour, hoping that the ultraviolet rays would take them away. Instead, I ended up with a horrendous second-degree burn on my face.

The pimples eventually went away on their own, but I was left with a scattering of small scars on my forehead. My father promised to take me to a plastic surgeon and have them taken care of, but somehow we never got around to it. When I became a plastic surgeon myself, I learned about chemical peels and dermabrasion, but I still didn't do anything about my forehead except hide the scars with makeup as best I could. It wasn't until I heard about CO_2 laser technology that I decided it was time to get rid of my scars. And while I was at it, I decided to do something about my eyes as well. The skin around them had developed fine crinkling as a result of all those days on the ski slopes and the beach sans sunglasses.

A dermatologist colleague of mine was just starting to perform laser resurfacing, so I asked her to do the honors. On the appointed day, I arrived in the operating suite and was asked to lie down on an examining table. Gauze pads were placed over my eyes, and I was cautioned to hold still. When I asked if the procedure was painful, the answer was reassuring: "Not bad. Kind of like rubber bands snapping against your skin."

Within minutes, however, I was in intense pain. Not being much of a stoic, I asked for a local anesthetic. I was even willing to inject myself if they weren't comfortable doing it. Finally another physician came in and gave me a local. It helped some but not much. Forty endless minutes later, the procedure was finally over. I may just have a low pain threshold (although many surgeons insist that laser resurfacing is not all that painful). All the same, I strongly recommend that if you are going to have this procedure done, insist on having intravenous sedation or general anesthesia.

At any rate, after my ordeal the doctor applied ointment to my face and gave me prescriptions for a painkiller and antibiotic. The first twenty-four hours were not bad. My skin oozed some and it would sting every now and then. I kept a basin of ice water by my bed so that I could dip a washcloth in it and drape the cool cloth over my face. That helped a lot, and I insisted on using it almost twenty-four hours a day for the first three or four days.

By the second day post-laser, my face was swollen, red, and crusty. I looked, frankly, awful. But by the fifth day, the swelling started to subside. By the seventh day, my skin was pink and smooth. It was beautiful, like the skin of a five-year-old, only pink. And the scars on my forehead? Gone. The crinkles around my eyes? Vanished without a trace. I was a laser convert.

CHEMICAL PEELS AND DERMABRASION

Although laser resurfacing has taken over as the main treatment for wrinkle removal, many surgeons still use chemical peels and dermabrasion to improve wrinkling or acne scarring in some individuals. (See Fig. 7.3.)

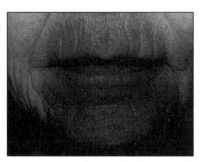 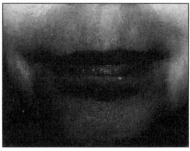

Photo credit: Carolyn J. Cline, M.D.

Figure 7.3 Before and after resurfacing with laser chemical peel or dermabrasion.

Chemical Peels

Chemical peels—especially light ones—are great for the skin and can help keep it looking refreshed. You do not have to see a plastic surgeon or dermatologist to get a chemical peel; many aestheticians provide them on a regular basis. Some older surgeons trained in the use of phenol peels still use them and obtain fabulous results. However, the phenol peel is unpredictable when not in the right hands and can give the skin an unnaturally pale appearance.

Dermabrasion

Dermabrasion mechanically removes some of the top layers of skin, more or less like sanding a piece of wood. This method is effective for treating depressed or pitted scars as well as wrinkles. An acne scar, for example, looks rather like a moon crater. If you were to shave down the mountain around the crater, the crater would be less noticeable. That, in essence, is what the surgeon does with a dermabrader.

Many doctors in my community treat upper lip wrinkles with the dermabrader. It's simple, quick, and easy, and the doctor doesn't have to buy a fancy expensive laser or rent one for a day. The only drawback with the dermabrader is that it can leave some lightening of the skin and hypopigmentary changes on the lip. Some women find this objectionable while others just cover it with makeup.

CHAPTER EIGHT

Men and Face-Lifts: Special Considerations

WHEN IT COMES TO AGING, men tend to have a better time of it than women. For one, they just don't seem to age as fast. This is partly because they have thicker skin, which doesn't tend to wrinkle as easily. Also, the skin on their faces and necks has a larger blood supply than a woman's, in order to nourish their growing beards. And, in our culture at least, age tends to enhance a man's power and status, while diminishing a woman's.

At least that's the way it has been until recently. Today, the emphasis on looking young seems to apply more and more to men as well as women, which explains why plastic surgeons are receiving more and more visits from men. In the early 1970s, men comprised perhaps 1 percent of all plastic surgery patients. In thirty years, the percentage has risen to 15 to 20 percent in some practices—maybe even higher in locations such as Los Angeles, New York, and San Francisco.

Regardless of the procedure(s) a man elects to undergo, his self-image and motivation are important factors in determining its success. The most perfect face-lift in the world may help a man feel better about himself but cannot be expected to change his life. Generally, men have different goals for plastic surgery than do women. Both seek plastic surgery to look more youthful and attractive. But for men, attractive means looking as masculine as possible. The desire to appear strong, courageous, bold, and aggressive has long been part of the male psyche, from the statues of the ancient Greeks and Romans to modern comic strip heroes such as Superman and Batman. In our image-conscious culture, men spend countless hours and dollars working to develop muscular, well-toned bodies. Plastic surgery is just an extension of this desire to look great.

The majority of male plastic surgery patients are between thirty and seventy years of age, although they tend to cluster toward the upper end of that range. As a rule, men tend to like the distinguished image that usually accompanies aging. It helps them in both business and their amorous conquests. A few gray hairs and well-placed wrinkles can be useful in the office and attractive on the dating scene. There are, however, some things about aging that men don't like—the biggest of these being hair loss and tired-looking eyes. That's why hair transplants are the most sought-after plastic surgery procedure for men, followed by eyelid lifts. Liposuction, face-lifts, and brow lifts are also increasingly popular among men.

This chapter will address some of the issues specific to men who are considering having hair transplants, face-lifts, or other anti-aging surgery.

HAIR TRANSPLANTS

Despite the success of such male sex symbols as Patrick Stewart and Yul Brynner, few men look forward to baldness. After attempts dating back at least as far as 5000 B.C., time and technology have come up with a fix (if not exactly a cure) for baldness. For men who are not helped by Rogaine or Propecia, modern hair transplant techniques offer a markedly better option than the telltale look of yesterday's hair plug transplants.

By far the most common cause of baldness is genetically determined male-pattern baldness, which is inherited from one or both parents. The male-pattern baldness, gene will be expressed only if normal levels of the male hormone testosterone are present in the bloodstream. The hair follicles around the sides and back of the head are not affected by the gene. This means that hair can be taken from these locations and repositioned in the bald areas where it will grow normally, thus eliminating the baldness.

Hair transplants can also be used to treat men or women whose hair is thinning in front due to various types of alopecia. A person who has generalized thinning all over the scalp is not a good candidate for hair transplantation, however.

Hair replacement surgery is also used to cover scalp defects that are due to either trauma or postoperative scarring. Sometimes I see patients interested in improving hair growth near a face-lift or brow lift scar. Scarring in this area often has a fair amount of tension that cannot be improved by scar revision. In such cases, hair grafts can provide good camouflage.

The least invasive and simplest hair transplant technique is micro or mini–hair grafts. The other techniques involve more or less extensive surgery on the scalp. In general, the healing phase for grafts is very short, and covering up the affected areas is relatively easy compared to a scalp rotation flap or tissue expansion.

Micro and Mini Grafts

Micro and mini surgical hair grafts are the most consistently successful treatments currently available for male-pattern baldness. They minimize scarring and provide long-term results that won't vanish over time. Also, the grafts' small size provides a natural appearance, alleviating the "corn row" or "doll's head" look that has long stigmatized hair replacement surgery. The skin must have a fairly good blood supply for the grafts to "take" properly.

The procedure is fairly simple and can be performed in the doctor's office under local anesthetic. The surgeon takes tiny grafts—

each containing one to five hairs—from the back of the scalp and places them surgically into the bald area using small incisions. Then the patient's head is wrapped in a turban and he is sent home. The following day the turban is removed, the grafts are cleaned, the hair is combed, and an antibiotic ointment such as Neosporin is placed on the graft sites. Over the next week, the small scabs around the graft sites fall off and the sites begin to look like small pinkish dots. Patients can return to work the next day, though most men wear hats until all the scabs have fallen off.

Over the next several weeks, the spots fade gradually into the scalp. About ten days after transplantation, the grafted hairs fall out. Within two or three months they start regrowing and continue to grow from then on. This technique can also be used to create or enhance eyebrows, and even eyelashes.

More Invasive Surgical Techniques

Other transplant techniques involve relocation of hair-bearing portions of skin to the bald area. One advantage of these various scalp flap methods is that, unlike micro and mini grafts, there is no interim hair loss stage. All involve more invasive surgery and extended healing periods, however.

Scalp Reduction and Scalp Extension   In a scalp reduction, the bald area is reduced by directly excising and removing some of the scalp skin. This is usually followed up at a later date with micro and mini grafts. For a scalp extension, a flat stretchy device is placed underneath the scalp skin to stretch the hair-bearing area. It is used in conjunction with scalp reduction in order to accelerate the rate at which bald areas can be excised.

The recuperation period for scalp reduction and scalp extension is similar. Once the procedure is performed, the sutures are typically removed in about ten days. In the meantime, you can wear a hat. Our patients are often able to style their remaining hair over the operated site and return to work.

Tissue Expansion   The tissue expansion procedure, which is less common today, has a longer recuperative period than the other methods. It is a more invasive procedure and usually requires intravenous sedation or general anesthesia. Tissue expanders are placed under the skin near the back of the scalp, extending from ear to ear. Once the incision has healed, the patient must return to the doctor's office once a week to have the expander inflated. After about eight weeks, the non-hair-bearing skin is excised and the expanded hair-bearing scalp tissue is advanced to cover the excised area. The main disadvantage of this method is that for several weeks the tissue expanders are large enough so that there is a noticeable difference in the size of the posterior scalp.

Scalp Rotation   For this technique, hair-bearing skin from the back and sides of the scalp is "rotated" to the front or anterior portion of the scalp.

FACE-LIFTS

Face-lifts are becoming an increasingly popular option for men wanting to "freshen" their appearance. Perhaps even more than women, men want a natural-looking result. They certainly don't want to look feminine, and they don't want the pulled-back look that shouts "I've had a face-lift." The best male candidate for a face-lift is one who wants to get rid of his "sad" look and droopiness around the neck area, as well as jowling along the jawline.

After a face-lift, men are more interested in a quick recovery with as little bruising as possible since they cannot wear makeup or hide the incisions with their hair. Men also have a higher tendency to develop complications from bleeding, or hematomas, because of the increased blood supply to the hair-bearing skin on their faces and necks.

Locating the Incision

When deciding where to locate a face-lift incision on a man, the surgeon must take into consideration the sideburns and hairline. The incision most commonly used goes around the sideburn, inside the ear near the tragus, around the earlobe, and back into the hairline. Some surgeons take the incision straight back into the hairline, while others place it along the hairline. You and your surgeon will have to decide which approach will work best.

The surgeon may also make an incision just underneath the chin to gain access to the area under the neck. This allows excess fat to be removed and the bands of muscle reworked and sewn to improve the appearance of the neck area.

BROW LIFTS

For men who are bald or losing their hair, choosing where to locate the incision for a brow or face-lift presents special challenges. For a brow lift, for example, you probably would not want to use the standard bicoronal incision. Instead, the incision could be placed inside an existing forehead crease. Another option is the direct eyebrow incision method. Endoscopic techniques may also be an option.

Heavy Forehead Wrinkling

If you have deep forehead wrinkles, the surgeon may weaken the frontalis muscle by transecting (cutting across) it during brow lift surgery. The frontalis, remember, is the muscle you use to raise your eyebrows, which also creates lines across your forehead. Weakening this muscle will reduce the creases.

In general, men tend not to be too concerned about forehead creases. They may even find them desirable because they represent strength and power, whereas women tend to want them removed. Just softening rather than eliminating forehead creases may be more appropriate for men.

Forehead Recontouring

We expect a man's brows to be more prominent than a woman's, but men whose brows are especially prominent may want to consider forehead recontouring. This involves trimming the bony tissue of the forehead to soften the "caveman" effect but without making it appear feminine. This is a specialized procedure and not all surgeons can perform it. You will need X-rays prior to surgery so that the surgeon can determine how much bone can be removed without injuring the sinus region, which is right underneath the brow bone.

EYELID LIFTS

After hair transplants, upper lid blepharoplasty is one of the procedures most commonly performed on men. The motivation for most men is professional, not aesthetic. Saggy, droopy lids can make a man look tired, and a perceived lack of energy is a handicap when it comes to getting promotions or sales. Though it might not be fair, good-looking people are perceived as more successful and therefore more desirable as employees or business associates. Several surveys have reported that substantial numbers of men would undergo cosmetic surgery if they felt it would improve their prospects for professional advancement.

Men also seek this type of surgery for functional reasons, primarily because the excess skin droops enough so that it impairs their vision. One man came to see me because his tennis game was not up to par. He was having a hard time returning the ball because he couldn't see it. He was a great candidate for blepharoplasty!

The Lower Lid

As we age, the fullness in our cheeks decreases as the fatty tissue under the skin is pulled down by gravity. This causes the cheeks to look flatter or even sunken, a condition called malar hypoplasia. At the same time, the skin of our eyelids gets thinner, and the fat underneath it becomes more prominent, which makes our lower lids look puffy. Consider Bill Clinton as an example. If you look at pictures taken during his governorship of Arkansas, he definitely had fuller cheeks. Now he has puffiness under his eyes and droopy cheeks.

We used to correct this puffiness by doing a lower lid blepharoplasty. Now, however, the trend is to perform a mid-cheek lift instead. In this procedure, remember, the entire cheek tissue is lifted off of the bony tissue of the middle part of the face. The tissue is then repositioned and secured. Often, especially if this procedure is being performed on an older individual, any excess slack that is elevated from the cheek region is treated by performing a temporal brow lift as well. (See Fig. 8.1.)

Mid-cheek lifts are discussed in chapter 5, and temporal lifts are discussed in chapter 6.

FACIAL IMPLANTS

Among men who have sought plastic surgery over the last couple of decades, rhinoplasty and chin contouring have been two of the most popular procedures. Over the past ten years the emphasis has

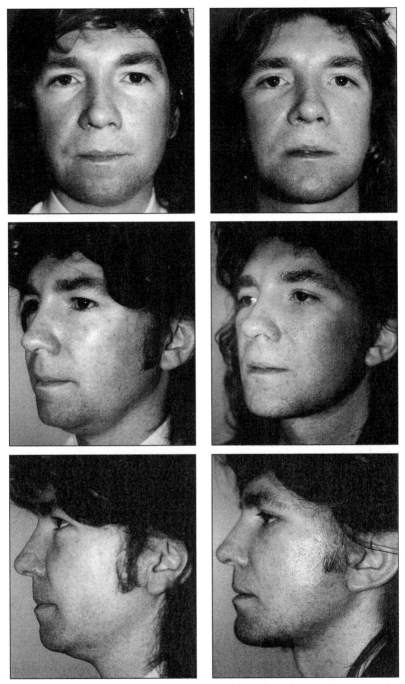

Figure 8.1 Male patient with SMAS face-lift and neck recontouring with chin implant. *Top*, front view before and after. *Middle*, three-quarter view before and after. *Bottom*, side view before and after.

increasingly been on altering the skeletal structure to meet the social demands for a strong, bold, masculine face—you know, that
rugged, chiseled jaw, Marlboro-man effect. The goal is to have a
strong angular appearance to the jawline and bold improvement in
the cheek area. Men seeking these kinds of changes will often bring
in pictures of male models from magazines such as GQ, just as
women will bring in pictures from *Vogue* to show how they want
their lips and eyebrows to look.

Previously, the only way to achieve those masculine facial forms
was through extensive craniofacial operations. The operations
achieved, at best, only some of the desired results and were potentially life threatening to boot. Now, however, we can accomplish
wonderful things using facial implants. Cheek implants can add a
healthy fullness and definition to the middle portion of the face and
are especially helpful for men with long, thin, drawn-out faces.
Chin implants are popular with men concerned about small,
feminine-looking chins or loss of definition along the border of the
mandible. One or both types of implants can be used to improve facial balance both in profile and three-quarter view.

Cheek and chin implants are discussed in detail in chapter 5.

MEN AS PATIENTS

By the time a man comes to see me for a consultation, he has for
the most part already made up his mind to have plastic surgery. I remember one man who said immediately after the consultation,
"Okay, when can I have the operation? Can I have it tomorrow?"
So, at least in my practice, once a man makes up his mind to do
something about his appearance, it doesn't take him long to follow
through. It's similar to when men go shopping for clothes, or anything else for that matter. They've made up their minds, bought the
merchandise, and left the store in less time than it takes most

women to decide what floor to go to first. I've also found that my patients tend to be men whose girlfriends or wives have had surgery with good results, and they want to try it for themselves.

It's a different story once they get to the operating room. As a group, men tend to be more anxious about plastic surgery than women. Younger men also tend to be slightly more anxious than older men (army veterans are quite calm!). I had one man who was so anxious about having surgery that he left the preoperative waiting area and walked all the way home. He later apologized and ended up having his surgery the following week with no problems.

In my own practice, I have found that men also tend to be somewhat more challenging patients with a lower tolerance for physical stress and lower pain thresholds than women. They usually require more medication than a woman undergoing the same procedure. They will be more agitated in the operating room and have a difficult time lying still. If you're a man considering having plastic surgery, you should consider having a board-certified anesthesiologist with you at all times who can provide some type of deep sedation or anesthesia to make you feel more comfortable.

The Recovery Period

Postoperative recovery is difficult for some men and easy for others. From my experience, men tend to tolerate changes in their appearance somewhat less easily than women, who are used to changing their hairstyle, makeup, and clothing. Men also have a greater challenge during the postoperative period because they cannot apply concealing makeup as a woman can.

Once men get through the initial two to seven days of recovery, however, they do very well. They tend to accept the healing process and realize, sometimes more easily than women, that plastic surgery represents improvement. Many women plastic surgery patients tend to be more critical, especially during the early phases of healing. Perhaps for this reason, men usually require less postoperative follow-up than do women.

Although men (as a group) are more open than women about plastic surgery in general, when it comes to their own surgery they prefer to keep it a closely guarded secret. Often the only person who knows is the "significant other" who accompanies them to the office and takes them home after their four- to six-hour ordeal. During the healing process they take refuge behind hats, beards, and sunglasses. They also are more reluctant to pose for before and after photographs.

As for the surgery and recovery period, men often find it's more arduous and uncomfortable than they had anticipated. I remember one man who was the CEO of several Fortune 500 companies. When I visited him in the recovery room, he gave me a look of pure misery and said, "I expected this to be like getting a haircut!" This was after a full face-lift, brow lift, and four-lid blepharoplasty, plus a tummy tuck from the day before! The first few days were kind of rough for him. Later he bounced back remarkably well, with a great attitude, and was quite happy that he'd had the procedure—but certainly not during the first seventy-two hours!

If you know how you feel during the first twelve hours of having the cold or flu, multiply that times three and you will have a fair idea of how you will feel right after the procedure. Fortunately there are new medications that can greatly decrease postoperative discomfort. As surgery goes, facial surgery is not that bad. Some patients don't even want to take post-op medication; they stick with plain old Tylenol after a face-lift.

Plan on having someone stay with you at least the first twenty-four hours. Stock your refrigerator with food that you like, though you should stick to saltine crackers or toast and 7-Up or ginger ale for the first day. If you have a recliner, that's where you will want to be. Most surgeons recommend sleeping with your head elevated for the first week or so and a recliner is perfect for this. A less desirable option is to pile extra pillows on your bed.

When Can I . . . ?

As soon as a man signs up for his face-lift, the next important question comes almost immediately. Actually, it's a two-parter: When can I go the gym and when can I have sex?

Here it is, guys: Following a face-lift, you should plan on not doing much of anything. For the first week, you are going to hang out at home and get the worst case of cabin fever you ever had! You'll watch Oprah Winfrey, *M*A*S*H* reruns, and maybe CNN and whatever old movies you can find. Even your well-stocked refrigerator will get pretty boring after a while, and you will be anxious to get out of the house and get on with your life. After the first week, you can go out, but you still need to take it easy. If you want a nice result, you'll need to follow your doctor's instructions, and that means rest, rest, and more rest.

Most plastic surgeons forbid their patients to engage in any type of sports activity for at least four to six weeks following surgery. This means any type of strenuous exercise such as aerobics, running, weight lifting, bike riding—and sex. I generally encourage patients to start a walking program. Walking, you say—how boring. Well, walking is a fabulous sport and if you walk for an hour straight (assuming you are up for it), you will get a nice, though low-key, workout.

The reason for these restrictions is that jogging, or going to the gym and bench-pressing 150 to 200 pounds could raise your blood pressure and you could develop some bleeding, or break a few sutures. Think about how great you will look in a few weeks and *follow instructions.*

Complications and How to Avoid Them

One of the most common complications following a face-lift, especially for men, is a hematoma, or collection of blood underneath the elevated skin flap. This is more common in men because of increased blood supply to the face. Also, men who are candidates for face-lifts are potentially at an age where hypertension, high blood pressure, and heart attacks can be of concern. This is why it is very important to make sure your blood pressure is under control and that you are in good health before having plastic surgery. Also, make sure you don't take any medications that contain aspirin or other ingredients that affect blood clotting for at least ten to fourteen days before having surgery.

Another reason men sometimes have problems is that they are more likely to overdo when they should be taking it easy after surgery. This is one time when you absolutely have to sit back and relax. Don't do *anything* for the first twenty-four hours except maybe push the buttons on the remote control or put cold compresses on your face. And don't do a whole lot more for the next several days. (If I sound repetitious here, it is because this bears repeating.)

If you are going to get a hematoma, it will usually happen within the first few days, most likely within the first twenty-four hours, after a face-lift. The main symptoms are increased swelling, pressure, and discomfort on one side of your face. *This is an emergency!* If you even suspect that you might have a hematoma, get it looked at right away, even if you have to call the doctor in the middle of the night.

If you do have a hematoma, it will be necessary for the surgeon to remove it. This is a relatively straightforward procedure. If it is a small hematoma, your surgeon may just aspirate it with a needle. Larger hematomas must be removed surgically. The surgeon goes back into the same incision, evacuates the blood clot, and then recloses the incision. As long as you are treated in time, the final result will not be affected. If you delay treatment, you may suffer some tissue loss, which can result in a lengthy healing process.

The second possible complication, although rare, is infection. This may show up as a pimple on your cheek. If you suspect an infection, check it out with your doctor as soon as possible so that it can be treated appropriately. Most surgeons administer antibiotics to their patients during surgery and send them home with more to take for a few days afterward. In my practice, I have seen two infections, and they were both on patients who had other surgeons do their face-lifts. This doesn't mean anything, except to show how uncommon they are.

A Final Warning: Smoking and Face-Lifts Don't Mix!

If you smoke at all, including the occasional cigar or even marijuana every now and then, give it up, especially if you are thinking at all about having a face-lift. If your girlfriend or wife smokes, kick her out of the house (at least whenever she is smoking)! Don't hang around friends who are smoking, either. The smoke causes constriction of the fine delicate vessels that provide the blood supply to your face—blood that you need in order to heal.

PART TWO

Once You Decide
to Proceed

Man has not yet finished being young,
when he is already starting to be old.
MARIO GONZALEZ-ULLOA

CHAPTER NINE

Designing the
Custom Face-Lift

So you've decided you are ready to do something about that person in the mirror. You meet all of the readiness criteria and you want to go ahead. How do you decide what exactly it is that you want done?

Any time a new patient comes to me for a face-lift consultation, I know it will be like no consultation I have had before. Each person presents a specific set of problems, which require a careful, section-by-section analysis aimed at designing a customized procedure or combination of procedures that will correct those problems *to the patient's satisfaction.* One person might need liposuction to remove neck fat, along with a face-lift. Another may need nothing more than eyelid lifts, or possibly a combination of an upper lid lift and cheek implants. Still another would benefit most by having liposuction and removal of excess skin plus a chin implant and tightening of the muscles underneath the chin followed later by laser resurfacing.

This design process should be a collaboration between surgeon and patient. While no surgeon should ever pressure a patient to have more procedures or more aggressive surgery than the patient wants, a good surgeon also has the experience and training to know what approach is likely to give a patient the best possible results. As I pointed out earlier, many people are so bothered by one particular problem, such as their necks, that they don't notice the changes that have been taking place on other parts of their face as well. A good surgeon will look at the face as a whole and may be able to suggest possible approaches that the patient might not have thought of, or even know about.

I've seen this happen numerous times in my practice such as when a patient in her late thirties or early forties comes to me wanting to have upper eyelid lifts. By the time the upper lids start to droop and sag, however, the lower lids are showing signs of age as well. More than once I've had patients insist on having just their upper lids done, only to turn around and wish they'd had the lower lids done as well. On the other hand, I've had patients insist that it is time for a face-lift when an eyelid lift and laser resurfacing may be all they would need to look great. So it's a good idea to at least listen to your plastic surgeon's suggestions and try to see your face the way he or she does before coming to a final decision.

I had a woman come to see me recently who said she had previously had her eyes done when she was forty-three. Now, ten years later, she just wasn't happy with the way she looked. When she looked in a mirror, she felt old. She wanted to feel refreshed but didn't know how to accomplish that. On examination, she appeared to have had the type of lower lid blepharoplasty we all performed ten years ago, where the fat was removed along with a little skin. Now she had a hollowness under her eyes that made her seem older. The skin was also wrinkly, like crepe paper. Nothing appealing about that, for sure! She also had quite a bit of sun damage from her early baby oil sunning days in the form of light and dark spots and wrinkles. Her neck contour still looked decent. She insisted she didn't want a face-lift, yet.

My recommendation for this patient was a full-face laser procedure to improve her aged skin, plus either a mid-cheek lift or cheek implants. Another possible option would have been a mini lift using a small incision just in front of her ear and tugging the cheek skin back toward the ear. However, this would not have addressed the hollowness from the previous lower lid blepharoplasty. She followed my recommendations and was delighted with the results.

As I mentioned earlier, sometimes the patient knows best. Patients can point, tug, and position their eyebrows like nobody else can. Having seen their faces a thousand times, they know exactly what it is that bothers them so much. Some patients, including me, actually design their own operations. When I am on the receiving end of plastic surgery, I have a plan all laid out. I practically draw the locations of the incisions so that the surgeon will know exactly what I want. It probably drives them a little nuts, I'm sure, but I get what I'm after. I got a taste of the same thing recently when performing liposuction on a woman's thigh. The patient wanted just one incision and showed me exactly where she wanted it, asking if it was doable that way. The answer, in her case, was a definite yes.

If a patient wants something that is not possible, then I definitely let him know and share my experience of what can be done instead. But patients often amaze me with their insight. One technique for doing butt tucks was actually instigated by a patient, who suggested to her plastic surgeon that the lift could be done through a small incision located in the buttock crease. The surgeon loved the idea, and worked with her to design an operation that has since given a number of patients the same beautiful results.

ANALYSES AND RECOMMENDATIONS

So that you can get an idea of how the design process works, the following figures (Fig. 9.1 through Fig. 9.9) contain pictures of potential plastic surgery patients along with my analyses of their faces and recommendations for giving each one the best "new look" possible.

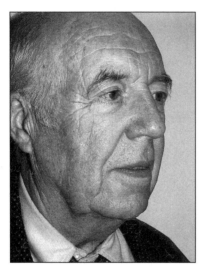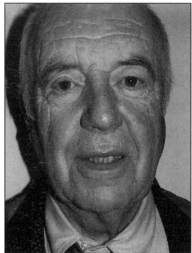

Figure 9.1 Seventy-three-year-old male (two views).

Patient #1

This is a seventy-three-year-old gentleman who is happy with his looks overall but would just like to have his skin checked every few months for skin cancer.

Analysis: Overall the patient could use some plastic surgery. There is evidence of aging in the eyes as well as the neck and jowl area. He doesn't really care much about these areas, however, and therefore would not be a good candidate for plastic surgery.

Recommended treatment: Nothing. However, if he gave us carte blanche we might gently recommend an upper and lower lid blepharoplasty and a face-lift and neck lift to improve these areas. Note: There is a difference between the position of the lower eyelids and this would be corrected during any type of eyelid procedure.

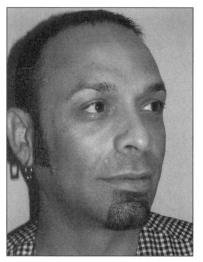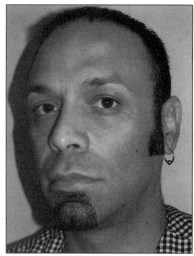

Figure 9.2 Man in his mid-thirties (two views).

Patient #2

This man is in his mid-thirties. He works as a hairdresser so he has to look at himself in the mirror all day, and he's not happy with what he sees. Mainly, he thinks he looks tired.

Analysis: The patient has prominent nasolabial folds and a cheek that is drooping. Also, his lower eyelid region is beginning to look puffy.

Recommended treatment: Either cheek implants or a combination of cheek lifts with or without implants. Another option is a lower lid blepharoplasty along with fat augmentation for his nasolabial folds and/or cheek region.

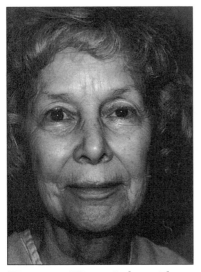 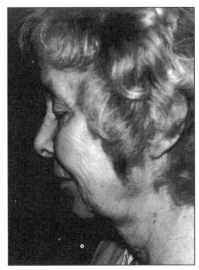

Figure 9.3 Woman in her mid-seventies (two views).

Patient #3

This patient is an ex–Eileen Ford model who is now in her mid-seventies. She's a wonderful lady and would love to look refreshed, but she doesn't want her friends to know that she's had anything done. (It's funny how many patients say exactly this. They want to look better, but they don't want anyone to know about it or recognize the improvement.)

Analysis: This patient has had no previous procedures and is showing the full signs of aging in her face from the top of her forehead to underneath her neck.

Recommended treatment: All parts of the face should be addressed at once to give her a nice balanced look. In this case, I would recommend a combination of a brow lift, a face-lift, and blepharoplasty for both upper and lower lids along with some lip augmentation and fine laser resurfacing to smooth out any wrinkling not corrected by the face-lift and brow lifts.

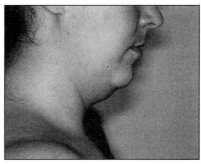

Figure 9.4 Thirty-four-year-old woman.

Patient # 4

This thirty-four-year-old patient wanted me to fix her neck.

Analysis: On examination she has evidence of fat and some excess skin underneath her neck.

Recommended treatment: Liposuction using three small incisions, one behind each ear and one underneath her chin.

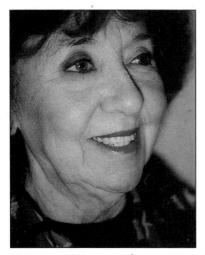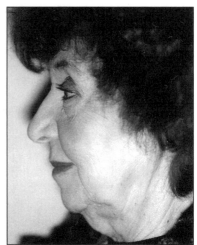

Figure 9.5 Woman in her seventies (two views).

Patient #5

This woman is in her seventies, but she appears older because her facial proportions are out of balance. She has an incredible vibrancy that transforms her, however, especially when she smiles!

Analysis: This is an example of a face that is not in balance because the chin is recessed.

Recommended treatment: A chin implant would greatly improve the facial lines and bring the face into balance. A full face-lift and upper and lower lid blepharoplasty would further enhance the beautiful aspects to match her incredibly vibrant nature.

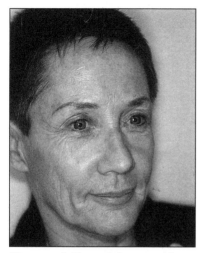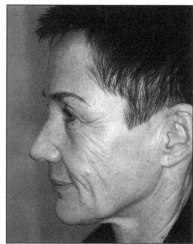

Figure 9.6 Forty-eight-year-old woman (two views).

Patient #6

This forty-eight-year-old woman wants to get rid of her wrinkles.

Analysis: The patient has deep frown lines and forehead wrinkles, and excess skin of the neck region and upper and lower eyelid regions.

Recommended treatment: Depending on the patient's wishes, this could be addressed with laser resurfacing and/or Botox injections, a brow lift, or face-lift procedures. In addition, upper and lower lid blepharoplasty procedures would also help.

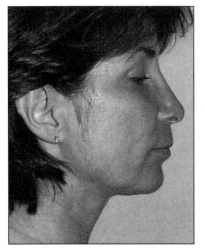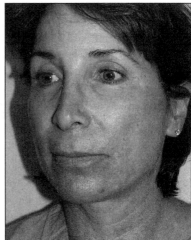

Figure 9.7 Woman in her mid-forties (two views).

Patient #7

This woman is in her mid-forties and has previously undergone an upper and lower lid blepharoplasty and a rhinoplasty. She would like some improvement in her appearance.

Analysis: While not quite ready for a lift, this patient is showing signs of aging underneath that could be addressed in the next several months or years. Currently her only concern is her skin tone and texture as well as some previous acne scarring on her cheek.

Recommended treatment: Full-face laser with Botox injections to preserve the effects of the laser plus some lip augmentation using collagen, her own fat, AlloDerm, or SoftForm implants.

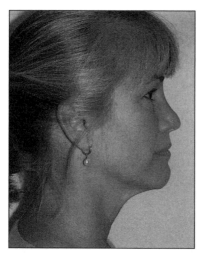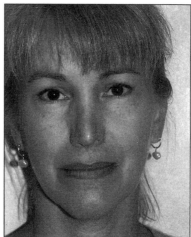

Figure 9.8 Forty-nine-year-old woman (two views).

Patient #8

This woman is just about to turn fifty, the big five-oh. Decades are dangerous years. They can make people feel frightened and uncomfortable. It's very common for plastic surgeons to see patients who are thirty-nine or forty-nine years of age.

Analysis: Overall she looks great. Her skin texture is excellent. To preserve it, I would recommend continuing with an excellent skin care regimen. The patient has previously undergone a rhinoplasty but would benefit from a touch-up procedure to improve the appearance of the tip, making it more balanced. The jawline is beginning to show some signs of aging, and she may want to address this sometime during the next few years. She is also showing some upper eyelid redundancy and some puffiness under her lower lids.

Recommended treatment: Repeat rhinoplasty, upper and lower lid blepharoplasty, perhaps liposuction underneath her jawline and in the neck region to remove some of the fullness underneath her neck, and/or early face-lift procedure.

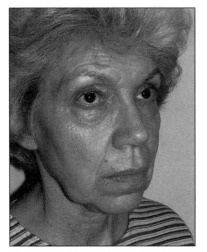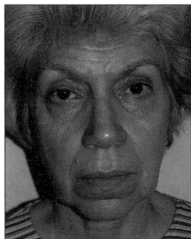

Figure 9.9 Author's mother (two views).

Patient #9

This is my mother, who for some unknown reason would never, ever consent to plastic surgery even though she says she can't stand the wrinkles on her face. The idea of a face-lift scares her tremendously, but one of these days she's going to go for a light laser resurfacing.

Analysis: On examination, she has very thick, olive skin with some fine wrinkling around her eyes and cheek region. Unlike her daughter, she doesn't have any excess fat underneath her chin.

Recommended treatment: Kid gloves for my mother. One of these days a full-face laser resurfacing, preferably with the CO_2, as the Erbium tends to be too gentle on the skin. Botox would be good but since it is less effective in patients over sixty she may need to have the injections repeated more frequently.

CHAPTER TEN

Choosing a Plastic Surgeon

ONCE YOU'VE DECIDED TO GO AHEAD with plastic surgery, the next step is to choose a surgeon—a decision that's right up there with choices such as jobs, homes, cars, and anything else that will have a major impact on your life. But how do you find the right plastic surgeon, one whose goals and expectations are compatible with yours, and who has the skills and expertise to give you the best results? This is a multistep process starting with careful research (such as reading this book) and culminating in professional consultations with the surgeons you are considering.

SURGEON QUALIFICATIONS

More physicians are calling themselves plastic surgeons these days than ever before. This is due largely to the increasing popularity of plastic surgery procedures. But it is also true that, in this age of managed care, many doctors see the potential for substantial profits in a specialty where nearly all patients pay up front and in cash. Specialists who are expanding their practices to include cosmetic procedures include ear, nose, and throat (ENT) doctors, dermatologists, and even dentists. Unfortunately, not all of these practitioners are properly trained as plastic surgeons. In some cases, their entire specialized training consists of weekend courses sponsored by equipment manufacturers or implant producers.

It may surprise you to learn that there are no laws regulating doctor training and qualifications beyond the requirements of state licensing boards. This means that anyone with a medical degree and a valid state license can call himself a specialist in any field of medicine he desires, including plastic surgery. So, doctors can advertise themselves as plastic surgeons without having studied the specialty sufficiently. Many such surgeons even claim to be "board-certified" in plastic surgery by the "Board of Cosmetic Surgery" or some similar-sounding organization. Be warned: these are unofficial organizations that are not recognized by the main governing board of the American Society of Plastic Surgeons (ASPS) or by the American Board of Medical Specialties.

The only truly board-certified surgeon is one who is certified by the American Board of Plastic Surgery (a member of the American Board of Medical Specialties). Board certification requires extensive training in plastic and reconstructive surgery, including at least five to seven years in the field performing a full range of reconstructive operations. This stands in sharp contrast to those self-proclaimed board-certified doctors who misrepresent their true expertise and training ability. Surgeons are considered board-qualified if they have been in practice for at least two full years and have taken and passed the board's written exams. To be certified, they must then pass an oral, or certifying exam. They are then granted board certification designating them as diplomates of the American Board of Plastic Surgery.

An ENT cosmetic surgeon is a physician who has had training in ear, nose, and throat surgery, plus one or two years of training in facial plastic surgery. ENT cosmetic surgeons are trained for face-lift, eye, and nose surgery only. By contrast, plastic surgeons have four years of general surgery training, followed by two to three years of plastic surgery training, and are qualified to perform most plastic surgery procedures. Some doctors further their education through added experience such as a fellowship, a three- to twelve-month training program either in a hospital or with an individual doctor. Plastic surgeons may also earn a CAQ (Certificate of Added Qualification) in hand surgery.

Table 10.1 explains the educational requirements for a doctor to specialize in plastic surgery.

It should be apparent that any doctors certified in plastic surgery have been highly trained in the specialty and that their practices have been evaluated by their peers. For the sake of your safety—and your appearance—stick with a bona fide board-certified surgeon.

Finding a Board-Certified Plastic Surgeon

The first step in your search for "Dr. Right" is to call the American Society of Plastic Surgeons for a list of recommended doctors in your area. You can request a doctor who specializes in one procedure, such as face-lifts, a doctor who is geographically desirable, a male or female, one who has operating privileges at your preferred hospital or surgery center, and so on. You should ask as many questions as possible since this will help to narrow down your choice of a doctor. Based on your criteria, they will probably give you three names along with postcards that you can mail to the physicians requesting that they send information or contact you directly regarding any procedures you are interested in.

Local and state medical associations are another good source of referrals. Many of them can provide brochures and other print materials listing names of surgeons as well as descriptions of certain procedures. Another great way to find a good plastic surgeon is to ask your family practitioner or other doctors whom you know and trust.

One of the best ways to find a surgeon is by word-of-mouth. If you know someone who has had a procedure you're interested in, and you like the results, ask her for the name of her doctor. Of course, you need to be diplomatic in your approach. If the person has not openly acknowledged her surgery, you probably won't win points by asking about it—quite the opposite. Just be ready with your questions in case she decides to open up! When it comes to patient recommendation, I also need to warn you that someone's experience with plastic surgery can be highly individual. One person

Table 10.1 Training of the Plastic Surgeon

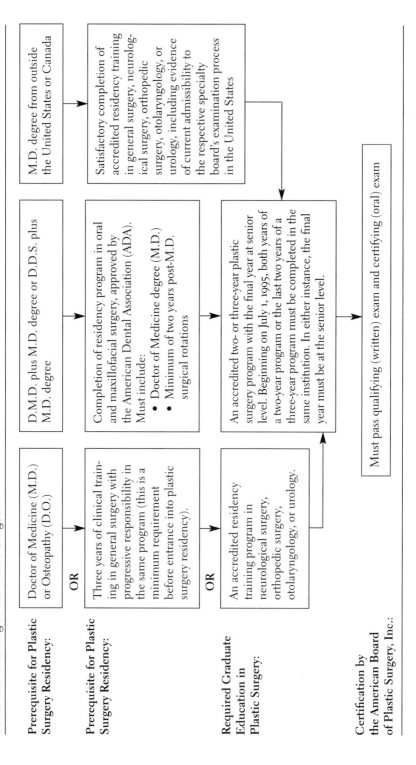

Prerequisite for Plastic Surgery Residency:	Doctor of Medicine (M.D.) or Osteopathy (D.O.)	D.M.D. plus M.D. degree or D.D.S. plus M.D. degree	M.D. degree from outside the United States or Canada
	OR		
Prerequisite for Plastic Surgery Residency:	Three years of clinical training in general surgery with progressive responsibility in the same program (this is a minimum requirement before entrance into plastic surgery residency).	Completion of residency program in oral and maxillofacial surgery, approved by the American Dental Association (ADA). Must include: • Doctor of Medicine degree (M.D.) • Minimum of two years post-M.D. surgical rotations	Satisfactory completion of accredited residency training in general surgery, neurological surgery, orthopedic surgery, otolaryngology, or urology, including evidence of current admissibility to the respective specialty board's examination process in the United States
	OR		
Required Graduate Education in Plastic Surgery:	An accredited residency training program in neurological surgery, orthopedic surgery, otolaryngology, or urology.	An accredited two- or three-year plastic surgery program with the final year at senior level. Beginning on July 1, 1995, both years of a two-year program or the last two years of a three-year program must be completed in the same institution. In either instance, the final year must be at the senior level.	
Certification by the American Board of Plastic Surgery, Inc.:	Must pass qualifying (written) exam and certifying (oral) exam		

may have had a terrific experience while another had a tough time recuperating, even though both had the same operation done by the same surgeon with the same cosmetic result.

THE CONSULTATION

Once you've narrowed the list of potential surgeons to two or three—or even one—the next step is to make an appointment for a consultation with each candidate. The initial consultation usually lasts about thirty minutes, but the amount of time will vary depending on the length of your discussions with the doctor and the doctor's schedule. Most plastic surgeons charge a fee for the initial consultation (average cost is $50 to $100), which could be the determining factor in how many doctors you plan to see. If you feel you can afford to see only one doctor, that's okay—unless you don't feel good about that doctor after the consultation. If that's the case, I urge you to consider the money well spent (after all, you found out you didn't want to use that doctor) and go visit someone else.

In essence, the consultation is a job interview and you are the interviewer. You want to make sure not only that the surgeon is qualified to do the surgery, but that he or she is someone you trust and feel comfortable with. At the same time, the surgeon will be evaluating you, your physical condition, and your expectations to see if you are, indeed, a good candidate for surgery. The consultation should include a discussion about your medical history. Be sure to tell the doctor about any illnesses you have had (or now have), any medications you are currently taking, those to which you may be allergic, and historically, any medications or procedures that you've had in the past. A complete medical examination will be done at another date, during your pre-op appointment.

This is the time to get *all* of your questions answered, even (or especially) the ones you think are silly or stupid. You may have read every brochure, pamphlet, and library book you could find about your procedure but still have questions about exactly what the doctor will do and how you will feel and look afterward. Or you may just as soon not know all the details about the procedure but still have questions concerning recovery time, potential complications, and expected results. The initial consultation is also the opportunity for you to ask questions about the doctor's qualifications including education, experience, and specialties. Most surgeons will have an album of before-and-after photos of previous patients that you can look through. This is a good way to see the doctor's work firsthand, and can also give the surgeon a chance to explain certain procedures.

It's a good idea to go prepared with a notebook with questions that you've written down about the procedure. Remember, you have a right to know everything the doctor will do to you, and the surgeon has an obligation to discuss your goals and expectations as well as any possible risks and complications.

Following are some of the questions you might ask the plastic surgeon at your first meeting:

1. *How long have you been in practice?* In this case, longer is not necessarily better. A surgeon with twenty years' experience will have seen more cases and have more experience dealing with complications. On the other hand, a younger surgeon is more likely to have been trained in the newest surgical techniques. Each may offer to you something that the other may not. You need to go with your "gut" on this one. In any case, the best gauge of competency is referrals and evidence of past results, such as patient references and before-and-after pictures.

2. *What procedures do you perform most frequently? How many cases of my type have you had in your career? How many in the past year?* Plastic and reconstructive surgeons receive training in both the cosmetic and the reconstructive aspects of their field, but many tend to specialize in one area or the other. For the purposes of procedures discussed in this book, you will probably want someone whose primary interest is in the field of facial cosmetic surgery

rather than, say, reconstructive hand surgery. This is not to say that a doctor couldn't be good at both, just that you want to make sure he or she has plenty of experience performing the procedures that you are interested in.

3. *Are you familiar with any of the new techniques? Do you incorporate them into your practice?* Again, this is not a cut-and-dried type of question. While new techniques may be improvements on older ones, some doctors are too willing to try relatively untested techniques out on patients. You want the right mix of openness to new ideas and concerns about safety and effectiveness.

4. *Do you have any before-and-after pictures that I can look at?* You want to be able to see what kind of work the surgeon has done before. It's especially helpful if you can see pictures of people with features and problems similar to your own.

5. *Can you give me the names of some former patients I can contact for references?* Some surgeons protect patient confidentiality by not allowing current or past patients to talk to prospective patients. Some doctors have staff members who have undergone the procedure you're interested in and who will be willing to speak with you.

6. *Are you in good standing with your state's licensing board? Are you board-certified? By what board?* Be careful with this question. If you have doubts, you can always check this out with the American Board of Plastic Surgery (see Resources).

7. *Are you associated with and on staff at a local hospital as one of their surgeons?* This question will eliminate most non-board-certified "cosmetic surgeons," as they are unlikely to be on a hospital's staff as plastic surgeons.

8. *What potential complications are involved with the procedures that I am interested in? Have you seen these complications before, and if so how did you handle them? Was follow-up surgery required?* Even though complications from facial plastic surgery are rare, they do occur. Your

doctor should give you details regarding any possible complications that could occur with the procedures you are
planning to have, as well as tell you how he or she would
handle them. You may also want to ask about the surgeon's
policy on touch-up or revisionary surgery. Many doctors
will do minor touch-ups free of charge, though you will
have to pay anesthesia and operating room fees, if required.

9. *Do you perform surgery in your office suite, and what types
   of surgeries are performed there? In which hospitals and
   surgery centers are you permitted to perform surgery?* If the
   doctor is permitted to perform surgery at one or more local
   hospitals, then you can (usually) safely assume that the
   hospital considers the doctor properly trained in those procedures. However, some doctors who have their own surgical suites can legally perform whatever procedure they
   wish without other doctors or hospital administrators
   watching them. In those cases, it's especially important for
   you to check out the doctor's qualifications, training, and
   experience.

10. *Do you perform the whole surgery or do you have an assis-
    tant help you?*

11. *Who will administer the anesthesia and what types are neces-
    sary?* If only a local anesthetic is to be used, the doctor will
    usually administer it. However, for procedures requiring in-
    travenous sedation or general anesthetic, you should have
    an anesthesiologist. Safety is my primary concern as a prac-
    ticing plastic surgeon. More than anything I want to provide
    patients with the safest environment possible. This is one
    reason I always use board-certified anesthesiologists rather
    than attempting to administer the anesthetic myself or have
    a nurse do it. I believe this is the only way to provide safe
    and effective anesthesia. Some patients are concerned
    about the extra expense, but as far as I'm concerned, having
    a qualified anesthesiologist is like having an insurance

policy. It's part of doing everything you can to make sure the procedure is as safe as possible.

12. *Do you conform to all of the guidelines for sterilization and infection control of OSHA (the Occupational Safety and Health Association)?*

13. *What are your fees?* Generally speaking, fees within a community will be pretty similar, although they may vary by area, with major metropolitan areas tending to fall on the upper end of the spectrum. Even if expense is a major issue for you, be careful about choosing a surgeon based on price alone. Having a face-lift is an expensive proposition, and you want to make sure your decision is made in an intelligent and well-thought-out manner. Be especially cautious about surgeons who advertise the lowest fees or who offer you a "bargain." As a consumer of plastic surgery, I would be suspicious of any surgeon who isn't in the same price range as his or her colleagues.

In addition to the above questions, you will want to get answers about issues that affect you, and not just a group of statistics. Here are a few more questions you might want to ask:

- Am I ready for this surgery, or should I wait a few years?
- How long will the results last? Will I have to have more surgery in a few years?
- Will I have scars? Where will they be? Will they fade over time?
- How painful will it be?
- Will I need to have someone take care of me afterward?
- When can I go back to work?

After your visit with the doctor, the patient coordinator will compile a surgical cost analysis that will either be mailed to your home or explained to you before you leave the office. This should include

the total surgeon's fee for performing the surgery, as well as esti-
mated hospital fees (including the cost of an overnight stay if
needed), surgery center costs, or fees for the doctor's in-office surgical suite. It should also include fees for the anesthesiologist's services, anesthesia and anticipated medications, plus fees for
additional services such as assistant surgeons, blood donation, laboratory work, and X-rays. Many patients prefer having this information mailed to them rather than discussing it at the office. That way
they have the opportunity to read and analyze the information at
home and not feel any pressure.

DECIDING WHICH SURGEON IS RIGHT FOR YOU

Once you have done your research and had consultations with one
or more doctors, you can analyze all the information and make your
decision. In addition to the answers you received, you will want to
consider more general impressions such as: How clean is the office?
How does the office staff make you feel? How does the doctor make
you feel? Did the doctor answer your questions and seem to understand your concerns? Is he board-certified by the American Board
of Plastic Surgery? If the surgeon recommended different or additional procedures from what you'd originally planned, do you feel
comfortable with the recommendations? Did you feel pressured to
sign up for surgery right away? If you did, forget this doctor and go
elsewhere. Plastic surgery is a personal decision, one that you make
alone. Your spouse or boy- or girlfriend cannot make it for you, and
the doctor certainly can't.

Make sure that you take all the time you need to feel comfortable with your decision. It may help to make a list of pros and cons
for each surgeon so that you can compare them. Sometimes a second visit to the surgeon you're considering helps you make up your
mind one way or the other. And trust your intuition — it is often the
best judge of what is right for you.

CHAPTER ELEVEN

Deciding Where to Have the Surgery

ONCE YOU HAVE MADE THE DECISION to go ahead, you and your doctor will need to decide where you will have the surgery. In addition to weighing the pros and cons of each type of facility, you should also consider details such as who will drive you there and bring you home, who will take care of your children or your office, and other issues you will need to deal with during the recuperation process. You may want to have your surgery done as close to home as possible (in a surgery center or hospital) or you may prefer to distance yourself from the turmoil of home life. Some people choose a surgeon in another state or even another country so that they can go through the initial healing period in private while all their friends and co-workers believe that they are off on a two-week vacation.

In the past, plastic surgery was performed only in hospitals or medical centers. However, surgery centers—where patients can be operated on as outpatients and released the same day—are becoming increasingly popular. A growing number of surgeons also maintain in-office surgical suites for procedures that do not require general anesthesia. Both of these options are considerably cheaper, and possibly more desirable, than hospitalization. This chapter discusses each option and its costs, benefits, and disadvantages.

THE SURGERY CENTER

Surgery centers are also called ambulatory or outpatient surgical centers. These freestanding facilities offer fully equipped surgical suites along with a staff of doctors, nurses, and technicians who perform various procedures on a same-day basis. Surgery centers offer a number of advantages over hospitals. First, as we have already mentioned, the cost is well below that of most hospitals for both patients and insurance companies—as much as 50 percent lower in most cases. Second, these centers usually provide patients with a pleasant, more intimate atmosphere where they can relax and feel more comfortable than they would in a hospital. Finally, a smaller, private facility is more conducive to visits from family and friends. Hospitalized patients often have to share rooms with one or more other people, which can restrict private conversations with visitors.

Most surgery centers charge an all-inclusive fee that covers:

- A medical history or examination
- Any necessary laboratory tests
- Room and equipment used for your procedure
- Most of the supplies used
- Any drugs administered to you
- Anesthesia
- Recovery room expenses

However, the fee for the surgery center usually does not cover:

- Your doctor's professional fees
- Any assistant surgeon's fees
- The anesthesiologist's fees
- Radiologist's fees, if needed
- Pathologist's fees, if needed

Surgery centers are often the preferred option for plastic surgery procedures that require general anesthesia (exceptions are discussed under the Hospital section on page 158). Make sure that you check with your doctor to see if he or she has operating privileges at a surgery center in your area. If you decide that hospital costs are prohibitive and using a center is the only way you'll be able to afford your surgery, and if your chosen doctor can operate only in a hospital, you may want to seek the services of another plastic surgeon who can offer you the advantages of a surgery center.

THE IN-OFFICE SURGICAL SUITE

These days, many plastic surgeons are able to offer patients the option of having surgery in a fully equipped and accredited operating room located in the surgeon's own offices. If available, this can be an ideal choice. The main advantages to an in-office suite are reduced cost, complete privacy, and a staff trained in and committed to caring for plastic surgery patients only. Although fees vary from one surgeon to the next, we can safely say that, on the whole, the in-office suite is the least expensive of the three options. Additionally, it offers the most comfortable, personal, and intimate way to have surgery. Another advantage is the fact that after surgery you can remain in the suite until you are ready to be driven home.

Most of the procedures described in this book can be performed in a fully accredited in-office facility. For patients who are older or of questionable health, however, we usually prefer a hospital setting. And let me amend the last sentence to say that if a patient has a questionable health history, such as a recent heart attack, heart disease, poorly controlled high blood pressure, diabetes, or is on blood thinners, I will not perform surgery unless an internist approves the procedure beforehand. Most internists would not approve surgery for such patients, except in special circumstances, and then the operation would be done in a very conservative manner. Generally speaking, however, 99.9 percent of our patients are healthy.

A word of caution if you are considering the in-office option: For your safety, make sure that the surgeon *and* the operating facility are fully accredited by the AAAHC. Accreditation means that the facility has undergone an intensive evaluation process that includes the rooms, equipment, and every member of the staff including physicians, nurses, and medical technicians. The accreditation process can take as long as six to eight months, and must be repeated every one to three years depending on the initial survey.

THE HOSPITAL

Having surgery in a hospital is by far the most expensive of the three options. A hospital stay means paying for a long list of services and equipment. It will probably seem as though every move you make, or that someone makes in your vicinity, is recorded by an invisible billing ghost who is lingering somewhere in your room. Here is a sampling of items you will be charged for:

- The room
- Operating room time
- Medications
- Intravenous solutions
- Dressings
- Lab work
- Anesthesia and equipment

Additionally, you will be billed separately by each physician involved in your surgery including your own surgeon, any assistant surgeons, and the anesthesiologist as well as the radiologist and pathologist, if needed (which is usually not the case in cosmetic cases).

In cases of medically required surgery, most of these charges are covered by health insurance carriers. However, because most cosmetic surgery is not covered by insurance, you will be responsible for all expenses. Most plastic surgeons require payment in full prior to surgery. Hospitals usually require a substantial deposit from patients whose insurance companies will not cover the surgery. They then bill you for any balance not covered by your deposit.

Not only do you get charged for more items in a hospital, but many of the individual costs are higher. For instance, the average operating room charge for a two-hour blepharoplasty (upper and lower eyelid surgery) was $935 in 1997. By comparison, the average operating room fee for surgery centers was $625 while the average fee for the in-office surgical suite was $375 for the same amount of time.

Another disadvantage of a hospital stay is lack of privacy. A registered nurse will pop in every few hours to check your vital signs, straighten your blanket, plump your pillows, and essentially, not leave you alone. As soon as you close your eyes and feel relaxation setting in, it will happen all over again.

Some plastic surgery procedures automatically require the patient to stay in the hospital for a minimum of one night, although that does not generally apply to the types of procedures discussed in this book. In these cases, the doctor will require you to have the surgery in a hospital or medical center. Some patients, however, prefer a hospital setting, particularly if they have underlying health issues or if they do not have anyone to care for them after the surgery. In the latter case, however, it would probably be cheaper (and more pleasant) to hire a private nurse to come to your home or to stay in a recovery center that specializes in caring for postoperative patients.

CHAPTER TWELVE

Getting Ready for Surgery

S<small>O YOU'VE DECIDED TO PROCEED WITH SURGERY!</small> Congratulations. You've taken that last look into the mirror and said this is it: Goodbye, wrinkles. Hello, smooth skin, younger neck contours, and a happier, more pleasant, and alert-looking face. Now what happens?

The first step is to decide when and where you'd like the surgery performed. The date will depend, of course, on the doctor's availability and your schedule. The time of day is more flexible. However, many patients prefer an early morning surgery so that they can wake up, go directly to the hospital, surgery center, or the doctor's surgical suite and not have to spend a long time feeling anxious about the procedure. Because you may not eat or drink liquids after midnight on the day before your surgery, it is best to schedule the procedure early in the morning whenever possible.

Next, you will need to decide where you would like to have your surgery performed—a hospital, a surgery center, or in the doctor's in-office surgical suite. After the patient coordinator has checked the surgeon's schedule and made the appointment for your surgery, she will verify the availability of the surgical location you have requested. Once this has been confirmed, you are on the way to your new look.

THE PREOPERATIVE APPOINTMENT

In our practice, once a patient is scheduled for surgery, we schedule a "pre-op" appointment approximately ten days to two weeks before the scheduled surgery date. The pre-op appointment usually lasts about thirty minutes, but a lot is accomplished during that time. First, it gives you and your doctor an opportunity to discuss expectations and concerns (both yours and the surgeon's), view before-and-after pictures, and discuss exactly what it is you want the surgery to accomplish. You may also get to meet staff members such as nurses and operating room technicians who will be involved with your surgery. You may even meet the anesthesiologist, if that person is available. (If not, the anesthesiologist should telephone you the night before and meet with you briefly the morning of surgery.)

During the appointment, the doctor should explain the procedure(s) in detail including the location of all incisions and the type of anesthesia to be used. With general anesthesia, you will sleep through the entire operation. With a local anesthetic, only the area to be operated on is numbed. A third and increasingly popular option is to combine local anesthetic with intravenous sedation, which will put you in a dreamlike state for the duration of the surgery. The choice depends on what type of surgery you are having, your doctor's opinion, and your personal feelings. Remember to have all of your questions about anesthesia ready for your doctor.

You probably will have thought of more questions about your procedure since you last saw the doctor, and this appointment is the time to get those questions answered. Remember, no question is off limits. It's your face and your money, and any doctor should be happy to answer any question that you ask.

Physical Examination

Before we are plastic surgeons, we are physicians concerned about your health. During the initial consultation, you and your surgeon briefly discussed your medical history. During the preoperative appointment, the surgeon will conduct a more detailed examination to determine how healthy you are and whether or not it is okay to proceed with the upcoming surgery.

Once again, be certain to mention any medications you are taking, any allergies, and any general health problems including heart or lung disease, cancer, high blood pressure, or bleeding tendencies. I have my patients fill out a health questionnaire that outlines their previous medical history, any prior operations, and current health problems such as high blood pressure, recent viral infections, HIV exposures, current medications, and current allergies. Certain medical conditions will probably exclude a patient from being a perfect candidate for plastic surgery. These include diabetes, uncontrolled hypertension, cardiac disease, recent heart attack, lung disease, emphysema, malnutrition, psychological instability, severe depression, severe obesity, and a history of smoking. However, some plastic surgeons will perform limited types of plastic surgery procedures on patients with some of these problems.

The majority of patients are healthy and most of our patients pass the physical exam with flying colors. If we have concerns about a patient's health, however, we will insist that he see his primary physician to determine whether there are any specific recommendations prior to proceeding with elective surgery.

Laboratory Tests

Prior to surgery your surgeon will also order some laboratory tests, which are typically done two or three days before the surgery date. This usually includes a complete blood count, urinalysis, and tests to check your blood clotting time. If you are over fifty or have a history of heart disease, an EKG will be ordered as well. Occasionally a chest X-ray will be ordered to rule out any lung disease, especially if you have a history of smoking. (P.S.: If this applies to you, quit smoking right now. It does not help with the healing process of a face-lift, or with any surgery, for that matter!) If there is a possibility that a patient could be pregnant or if she is of child-bearing age (sometimes face-lifts are performed on patients in their late thirties or early forties), a pregnancy test will also be ordered.

Before Pictures

The next step in the pre-op appointment is taking the "before" pictures so that they will be ready by the day of surgery. Often patients can't believe the pictures ("Do I really look like this? I'm glad I'm here!"). All plastic surgeons take before pictures prior to performing any procedure. This helps both the surgeon and you because it helps to compare what your face (or body) looks like in two dimensions. When you look at a face in three dimensions, shadows and contours may make it difficult to see the irregularities that you or the surgeon are concerned about.

Often surgeons tack up the before pictures in the operating room to serve as a guide during surgery: "Maybe I need to take more off the right side than the left side . . . the fullness is worse on the left side . . . the right eyebrow needs to be repositioned more than the left." After the operation, and during the healing process, we use the before pictures to help evaluate the results. How much improvement have you had? Did we correct everything that we wanted to? If not, what can we improve on? Despite our efforts to make everything as perfect as possible, sometimes the body just doesn't heal the way you would like it to. Sometimes, albeit rarely, a "touch-up" may be called for. This will be discussed with your plastic surgeon sometime during your recovery when you are healing, if in fact it is necessary at all.

Pictures also provide a great educational tool for patients, as well as for helping them get through that difficult, initial postoperative period. During the healing process, bruises become evident and people wonder if they'll ever get better. This is the time we bring out the before pictures so they can see that, yes, there is a difference.

The before-and-after pictures remain part of your medical record and thus confidential, unless you give permission for your pictures to be viewed by other patients who may be considering the same type of surgery.

Someone to Watch Over You

Not that long ago, I performed a face-lift on a woman who informed me in the recovery room, after the operation, that she had no one to take her home and take care of her. Well, we tell all of our patients during the pre-op appointment that they will need a licensed driver to take them home and be with them for at least twenty-four hours, especially if the surgery involves anesthesia. Guess she missed that part. . . .

Actually, this is not an uncommon problem, and it happens frequently in my practice. These days many people are too busy to develop friendships—their work schedule is too heavy, life is too hectic, kids are the main focus besides work, and so on. More to the point, most people consider plastic surgery very private—pretty much a matter for you, your mirror, your plastic surgeon, and nobody else. If you have a loyal spouse, or a friend who has been through the same thing, you might feel comfortable asking, "Hey, can you pick me up afterward and stay with me?"

If not, you need other options. In our practice, we refer patients to a registered nurse, LPN, or medical assistant who can be with them for twenty-four hours, or longer as needed, following surgery. Fees vary but they generally range from $175 to $350 per night. Like the anesthesiologist, it's well worth it. You will not have plastic surgery often—maybe only once or a very few times in your life. It is necessary that someone take care of you.

Consent Forms

After any photography is completed, you will meet with the doctor's patient coordinator to sign consent forms and discuss financial arrangements. In most cases, you will be required to sign both a general surgical consent form and a financial agreement form.

The surgical consent form verifies that you recognize and understand completely the nature and consequences of your procedure(s), with certain points mentioned and listed as having been specifically made clear. By signing the form, you agree that your doctor has explained the procedure, risks, and any complications that may occur.

The financial agreement form will state something along the lines of, "The practice of medicine is not an exact science; fees paid are for the performance of the procedure(s) only, and not a guaranteed result. Although a good outcome is expected and every effort has been made to establish realistic expectations, there cannot be any warranty, expressed or implied, as to the results that may be obtained. Problems relating to, or complications from, your surgery may result in additional costs to you. These costs may include additional anesthesia and facility fees, hospital costs, physician's fees, or other specified charges."

You may be asked to sign a photography consent form. This acknowledges that photos can be taken at any time during your procedure but only with the permission of your doctor. It also gives the doctor permission to publish photos and information relating to your surgery in newsletters, books, and journals, but without identifying you by name.

Once you have signed these documents, they are witnessed and considered legal and binding. If you are uncomfortable about any part of a form, be sure to discuss it with the patient coordinator or the doctor before you sign.

Payment

After your initial consultation with the doctor, you will have received a cost breakdown for your surgeon's fees, as well as those for any assisting doctors and the hospital or surgery center. Most plastic surgeons require payment in full for any cosmetic or elective surgery at the pre-op appointment. So make sure that you've brought your checkbook, credit card, cash, or money order with you for payment at this appointment. Financial arrangements are discussed in chapter 16.

Instruction Booklet

Before patients leave the office, we give them a personalized booklet that summarizes what they need to know about their surgery including:

- What medications to avoid
- What to do the night before surgery
- Specific instructions related to the procedure(s) they are having done
- Possible complications from the procedure(s)
- Expectations
- Postoperative instructions

The material is intensive and very thorough. We have patients read and initial a copy of each page before leaving the office. Then they take their booklet home to keep for reference.

If you are having surgery at a hospital, you will also receive a preadmission packet. This will include general information for patients explaining the important preadmission appointment at the hospital, information on hospital charges, insurance, and deposit requirements. You will also receive a patient instruction sheet with further information about the preadmission appointment, things to remember on the day of your surgery, advice about what clothing to wear, and a reminder to leave valuables at home and to make a list of any medications you are taking. The hospital will require that a responsible driver take you to the hospital and drive you home afterward. They will also want copies of your lab results.

Patients are usually asked to call the hospital within seventy-two hours prior to surgery to schedule the preadmission appointment.

At this appointment, you will preregister, have any lab work done, receive further pre-op instructions, review your health history, and answer any questions.

GETTING YOUR BODY READY FOR SURGERY

It is important that you be as healthy as possible prior to your surgery. The healthier you are, the faster you will heal, and the less likely it is that you will have complications. The three most important factors to consider are nutrition, avoiding medications that can interfere with the blood-clotting mechanism, and smoking.

Nutrition

To ensure proper healing and tissue repair, your body needs to get all the protein, calories, vitamins, and minerals that it can. The nutrients in food can strengthen your immune system and, therefore, help prevent postoperative infection.

Adequate protein is needed to form new skin cells to cover the surgical wound and, with calories, help white blood cells to function properly and fight bacteria. Protein is found in foods such as meat, poultry, fish, eggs, beans, and nuts. Calories are also needed to ensure that several important repair processes occur.

Vitamins and minerals are important both for repairing tissue and for increasing your resistance to infection. Some of the most important vitamins are C and A. Foods rich in vitamin C include citrus fruit, tomatoes, bell peppers, potatoes, cabbage, and broccoli. Vitamin A is found in foods such as milk, egg yolks, and liver. A nutrient that the body converts to vitamin A is beta-carotene, which is found in orange-yellow and dark green vegetables and fruits such as sweet potatoes, winter squash, carrots, apricots, cantaloupe, and spinach. Some doctors recommend taking extra doses of vitamin C for two weeks prior to surgery along with vitamin E, which is known to aid in healing.

Important minerals for healing include iron and zinc. Good sources of zinc include oysters, wheat germ, beans, beef, and milk, while iron can be found in foods such as liver, red meat, poultry, beans, prunes, and iron-fortified cereals and breads. If a patient is low in potassium, the doctor will often recommend supplements of it as well.

If you haven't been eating a healthy variety of foods, it's a good idea to begin a new nutrition program to ensure that your body is ready for surgery. The U.S. Department of Agriculture recommends these daily guidelines:

2 to 3 servings from the milk, yogurt, and cheese group
3 to 5 servings from the vegetable group
6 to 11 servings from breads, cereals, rice, pastas
2 to 3 servings of meat, poultry, fish, beans, eggs
2 to 4 servings from the fruit group

Besides eating properly, remember to use fats, oils, and sweets sparingly, drink lots of water, and get plenty of rest.

Avoiding Problem Medications

During our preoperative appointment with patients, and this includes both men and women, a surgeon will discuss the importance of staying off particular medications such as aspirin, ibuprofen, Motrin, Advil, and any product containing aspirin that may affect the blood's ability to clot. (Table 12.1 provides a list of all aspirin-containing products that can affect bleeding and the overall plastic surgery operation.) Our blood contains special cells called platelets that aid in the clotting process. Many aspirin products and anti-inflammatory medications affect platelet function, which in turn harms the blood-clotting mechanism. This can lead to bleeding problems. For this reason, most surgeons ask patients to avoid taking any such medications for ten days to two weeks preceding surgery.

Table 12.1 Medications to Avoid Before and After Surgery

If you are taking any medications on this list, they should be discontinued ten days prior to surgery. Only Tylenol should be taken for pain. All other medications that you are currently taking must be cleared specifically by your doctor and the nursing staff prior to surgery. *This is absolutely necessary!*

Aspirin Medications to Avoid

Acetilsalicylic Acid
Adprin-B products
Alka-Seltzer products
Amigesic
Anacin products
Anexsia w/Codeine
Argesic-SA
Arthra-G
Arthriten products
Arthritis Foundation
  products
Arthritis Pain
  Formula
Arthritis Strength
  BC Powder
ASA
Asacol
Ascriptin products
Aspergum
Asprimox products
Athropan
Axotal
Azdone
Azulfidine products
B-A-C
Backache
  Maximum Strength
  Relief
Bayer products
BC Powder
Bismatrol products
Buffered Aspirin
Bufferin products
Buffetts II
Buffex
Butal/ASA/Caff

Butalbital
  Compound
Cama Arthritis
  Pain Reliever
Carisoprodol Compound
Cheracol
Choline Magnesium
  Trisalicylate
Choline Salicylate
Cope
Coricidin
Cortisone Medications
Damason-P
Darvon Compound-65
Darvon/ASA
Dipentum
Disalcid
Doan's products
Dolobid
Dristan
Duragesic
Easprin
Ecotrin products
Empirin products
Equagesic
Excedrin products
Fiorgen PF
Fiorinal products
5-Aminosalicylic Acid
4-Way Cold Tabs
Gelpirin
Genprin
Gensan
Goody's Extra Strength
  Headache Powders
Halfprin products
Isollyl Improved

Kaodene
Lanorinal
Lortab ASA
Magan
Magnaprin products
Magnesium Salicylate
Magsal
Marnal
Marthritic
Meprobamate
Mesalamine
Methocarbamol
Micrainin
Mobidin
Mobigesic
Momentum
Mono-Gesic
Night-Time
  Effervescent Cold
Norgesic products
Norwich products
Olsalazine
Orphengesic products
Oxycodone
P-A-C
Pabalate products
Pain Reliever Tabs
Panasal
Pentasa
Pepto-Bismol
Percodan products
Phenaphen/Codeine #3
Pink Bismuth
Propoxyphene
  Compound products
Robaxisal
Rowasa

Table 12.1 *Continued*

Aspirin Medications to Avoid, continued

Roxeprin	Sodium salicylate	Tricosal
Saleto products	Sodol Compound	Trilisate
Salflex	Soma Compound	Tussanil DH
Salicylate products	St. Joseph Aspirin	Tussirex products
Salsalate	Sulfasalazine	Ursinus-Inlay
Salsitab	Supac	Vanquish
Scot-Tussin Original	Suprax	Wesprin
5-Action	Synalgos-DC	Willow Bark products
Sine-Off	Talwin	Zorprin
Sinutab	Triaminicin	

Ibuprofen Medications to Avoid

Actron	Haltran	Nuprin
Acular (ophthalmic)	IBU	Ocufen (ophthalmic)
Advil products	Ibuprin	Orudis products
Aleve	Ibuprofen	Oruvail
Anaprox products	Indomethacin products	Oxaprozin
Ansaid	Ketoprofen	Piroxicam
Cataflam	Ketorolac	Ponstel
Clinoril	Lodine	Profenal
Daypro	Meclofenamate	Relafen
Diclofenac	Meclomen	Rhinocaps
Dimetapp Sinus	Motrin products	Sine-Aid products
Dristan Sinus	Nebumetone	Sulindac
Etodolac	Nalfon products	Suprofen
Feldene	Naprelan	Tolectin products
Fenoprofen	Naprosyn products	Tolmetin
Flurbiprofen	Naprox X	Toradol
Genpril	Naproxen	Voltaren

Table 12.1 Medications to Avoid Before and After Surgery, *continued*

Other Medications to Avoid

A-A Compound	Flagyl	Pyrroxate
A.C.A.	4-Way w/Codeine	Ru-Tuss
Accutrim	Fragmin injection	Salatin
Actifed	Furadantin	Sinex
Anexsia	Garlic	Sofarin
Anisindione	Heparin	Soltice
Anturane	Hydrocortisone	Sparine
Arthritis Bufferin	Isollyl	Stelazine
BC Tablets	Lovenox injection	Sulfinpyrazone
Children's Advil	Macrodantin	Tenuate
Clinoril C	Mellaril	Tenuate Dospan
Contac	Miradon	Thorazine
Coumadin	Opasal	Ticlid
Dalteparin injection	Pan-PAC	Ticlopidine
Dicumerol	Pentoxyfylline	Trental
Dipyridamole	Persantine	Ursinus
Doxycycline	Phenylpropanolamine	Virbamycin
Emagrin	Prednisone	Vitamin E
Enosaparin injection	Protamine	Warfarin

Tricyclic Antidepressant Medications to Avoid

Adapin	Endep	Pertofrane
Amitriptyline	Etrafon products	Protriptyline
Amoxapine	Imipramine	Sinequan
Anafranil	Janimine	Surmontil
Asendin	Limbitrol products	Tofranil
Aventyl	Ludiomil	Triavil
Clomipramine	Maprotiline	Trimipramine
Deipramine	Norpramin	Vivactil
Doxepin	Nortriptyline	
Elavil	Pamelor	

If you have taken medications that could affect blood clotting during the two weeks prior to surgery, be sure to tell your doctor. She may be able to order a special test called a "bleeding time," which helps determine whether your platelets are functioning properly. If your bleeding time is normal (anywhere from two-and-a-half to nine-and-a-half minutes), surgery can proceed.

Smoking

Most plastic surgeons ask patients who smoke to stop for at least two weeks prior to, and at least two weeks after, surgery. Some simply refuse to operate on patients who smoke. The reason for this is simple. The nicotine in cigarettes or cigars causes the tiny blood vessels to constrict. Without an adequate blood supply, the skin dies and turns black, causing a serious condition known as skin necrosis. Patients undergoing face-lifts run the greatest risk of skin necrosis because the skin of the face depends so much on small blood vessels for its blood supply. It may not be enough to stop smoking, either. Secondary smoke can also create a hazard.

If you know that you will have difficulty quitting smoking, postpone plastic surgery for the time being. Consult with your family doctor, ask for the latest in nicotine patches, and quit. Reward yourself with plastic surgery when you succeed. It will be well worth it.

CHAPTER THIRTEEN

The Day of Surgery

Y OU'RE ALL SET. YOU'VE MADE ARRANGEMENTS for childcare and
time off from work, cleaned your house, stocked the refrigerator, and maybe laid in a supply of videos or paperback novels.
You've let your spouse, family, or significant other know that you
will be "out of service" for the next week or so, and that you would
appreciate any extra support they can provide. Now it's time to get
ready to go. You've followed your doctor's instructions to the letter,
including:

1. You've stopped smoking, eaten nutritious meals, avoided aspirin and other "forbidden" drugs, and gotten plenty of rest
   for the last couple of weeks.
2. You've had nothing to eat or drink since midnight except a
   tiny bit of water needed to swallow the pill you were in-
   structed to take an hour or so before your scheduled appointment. This is a mild sedative, such as Halcion, that will
   help you feel calm and drowsy. (If you are having surgery at
   a hospital or surgery center, you may not receive the pill
   until you arrive at the site.)
3. You've taken a bath or shower to minimize the chance of
   infection, and you are not wearing any makeup.
4. You're wearing loose, comfortable clothing that can be removed easily and put back on after surgery, and that doesn't
   have to be pulled over your head. An oversized button-front
   shirt is ideal.

5. You've taken off all of your jewelry (including earrings and wedding ring) and made sure you don't have any valuables in your purse or pockets.

6. You have your completed medical and insurance forms (unless they have already been filled out and turned in).

7. You've arranged for an adult to be at the hospital or surgery center during the surgery and to drive you home and stay with you for the first day, or you've made arrangements to be taken to a recovery center or retreat.

8. You've filled any prescriptions given to you by the surgeon or your regular doctor.

Now your "designated driver" is waiting to take you to the doctor's office, surgery center, or hospital. If you're like most patients, you're feeling somewhat nervous but also relieved that the long-awaited day is finally here. What can you expect? Your day will probably go something like this:

AT THE SURGERY SITE

Depending on where you are having your surgery, you will probably be asked to arrive an hour to an hour and a half before the time scheduled for your operation. When you arrive at the surgery location, you hang up your coat and settle in with a magazine on a comfortable couch. Often when a patient is scheduled for an in-office procedure, the doctor's staff will not schedule other patients to be in the waiting area at the same time. The whole objective is to make the patient as comfortable and relaxed as possible. If you are at a surgery center or hospital, you may be asked to complete some last-minute paperwork, such as consent forms.

We generally ask our patients to arrive around 7:30 A.M. When they arrive, they are signed in and asked to verify who will be taking them home. We also double-check to make sure they have not had anything to eat or drink since midnight. Having anything in your stomach before an anesthetic is administered can be dangerous because of the possibility that you might aspirate (inhale the stomach contents into your breathing passages). I remember one patient who had orange juice and a bagel prior to her arrival. Unfortunately we had to send her home and reschedule her surgery for a later date.

Between 7:30 and 8:00 A.M. the operating room staff, anesthesiologist, and I meet with the patient. This gives the patient an opportunity to ask any last-minute questions and make any requests for additions or changes to the planned procedures. Often, for example, a patient will add an extra site for liposuction, or ask us to remove a mole that she forgot to mention during the pre-op appointment. This is also the time to report any health changes since your pre-op appointment such as a cough or a cold.

Next comes the preoperative marking. For a face-lift, the best way to mark someone is in the sitting or standing position. This is because the lines of the face change when you lie down. Each surgeon has his own approach to face-lift markings. I usually prefer to have the patient in a sitting position. Using a surgical marker, I outline the areas I will be working on. For example, if the patient is having a face-lift, I mark any and all deep creases such as those on the forehead, the area around the mouth, and the bands of tissue underneath the neck. I also outline any pockets of fat I want to remove and/or reposition during the procedure.

By this time you should be feeling a little groggy from the sedative. You will be taken into a room where an assistant will help you undress, put on a gown, and store your purse and other belongings. These days, most patients having cosmetic surgery walk to the operating room although some hospitals may require you to be brought in on a gurney. Once in the operating room, expect it to be rather chilly. Operating rooms are generally kept very cool because of the heat from the operating room lights above. The staff will give you blankets and do whatever they can to make you feel as

comfortable as possible. In our operating room, we have music for
our patients to listen to while we make all final preparations. This
includes attaching instruments to monitor your blood pressure,
heart rate, and blood oxygenation, and washing the areas to be operated on with an antiseptic solution. At the same time, the anesthesiologist will be inserting an intravenous catheter into your arm
or hand for administering the anesthesia or sedation.

If you are having a general anesthetic you'll be asked to count
backwards from one hundred. You'll start to feel a little woozy . . .
and the next thing you know someone will be greeting you in the
recovery room to let you know it's all over. If you have intravenous
sedation, you will be dreamily aware of activity going on around you
for what will seem like a fairly short time . . . and then you'll wake
up in the recovery room. If your surgeon is using local anesthetic
only, you will be pretty much wide awake throughout the whole
thing. I personally prefer intravenous sedation or general anesthesia for most procedures because I want my patients to be as comfortable as possible. Not to mention the fact that a squirming,
wriggling patient makes my job a lot tougher! Seriously, though, I
cannot emphasize enough the importance of having an anesthesiologist present. Don't be talked into saving a few dollars on the
anesthetic. Some doctors will provide the anesthetic themselves or
have a nurse provide it. Personally, I don't think that this is as safe.
In our office we provide a board-certified anesthesiologist for all of
our cases. That way, patients have two highly qualified doctors taking care of them at all times while they are in the operating room.

IN THE RECOVERY ROOM

You will probably feel a little groggy when you wake up. If you had
general anesthesia, you may feel cold as well, but someone will be
there with lots of blankets to keep you warm. You may also have a sore
throat. This is because the anesthesiologist inserted a tube after you

were asleep in order to keep your airway open and ensure an adequate flow of air. The soreness dissipates fairly quickly. You may also be thirsty. The nurses will probably offer you ice chips or 7-Up to soothe your throat and relieve your thirst. You may experience some nausea, but with today's modern anesthetics this is fairly unusual.

Depending on the type(s) of surgery you've had and your surgeon's preferences, you may or may not have some sort of dressing over the incisions. You may also have drains behind one or both ears to help collect any fluid that builds up under the skin flaps. Both dressings and drains will be removed in a day or two when you go back to the doctor. If you've had your eyes done, you may have ice packs on your eyes. However, if you've had a face, brow, and/or cheek lifts, it's important not to put any ice on your face itself, especially the cheek region.

About an hour to two hours after you wake up, you will be through the recovery phase and ready to go home or to a recovery center or retreat, if that is what you have chosen. If the operation is done in the hospital, you will be taken up to your room to spend the night.

AT HOME . . . THE FIRST DAY

You'll probably still be feeling rather "out of it" on the way home. Some of my patients can't even remember the car ride home after the operation. Once home, most patients are relieved and glad to have the whole thing over with. Your driver will help you out of the car, into the house, and possibly to the bathroom. Remember to walk slowly, avoid sharp turns and movements, and aim yourself in the direction of the bedroom or wherever you'll be spending your recovery time.

It's a good idea to have your lounge outfit or pajamas ready and waiting on your bed or recliner. The first few hours are usually spent lying down with your head elevated. A recliner is perfect for this, but if you don't have one you can make do by piling extra pillows under your head. If you've had eyelid surgery, ice packs—or bags of frozen peas—can help keep down pain and swelling. Just don't put them on your face; put them on your eyelids only.

Your attendant can help you lie down, pull up the covers, plump up your pillows, and place your pain medication and water within easy reach along with a clock so you know when to take your pills. You may also want other supplies nearby such as tissues, crackers, ginger ale or 7-Up, and the television or stereo remote control. If you are feeling at all queasy, you may also want a small pan or basin close by in case you get sick. Having the telephone close by is appropriate in case your doctor calls to check up on you. You may also want your postoperative instruction booklet next to you so that you can refer to it as needed.

If you are hungry or thirsty, ask for whatever you'd like unless your surgeon has given you specific dietary restrictions. However, you should not drink any alcoholic beverages or take any medicine not prescribed by your doctor. You'll also want to keep it light for the first twenty-four hours since rich, heavy foods might make you feel nauseated. Most people's stomachs tend to be on the sensitive side for the first twenty-four hours, and you'll probably want to stick to 7-Up or ginger ale with saltine crackers or toasted white bread. If you've received cheek or chin implants, you will probably be on a clear liquid diet, with careful use of mouthwash afterward. After the first twenty-four hours, most patients can resume their normal diet.

Your job now is to simply lie back and rest, and your attendant's job is to help you do that. Very few people feel like carrying on any kind of a conversation during this period. They mostly just want to be left alone. You can watch television, listen to music, or just close your eyes and do nothing. You need all of your energy to heal. If possible, young children and pets should be elsewhere for at least the first day or two. It's especially important to keep cats away from you and your bed during the healing process because they carry oral organisms that can cause problems with infections.

Pain and Discomfort

Depending upon which procedure(s) you've had done, you may experience some discomfort after the anesthetic has worn off. Most doctors provide pain pills or prescriptions to help with any postoperative pain. Unless you've had eyelid surgery, you should avoid ice packs and heating pads since they can bruise newly moved tissue. You will probably have little or no pain after a face-lift or eye surgery, but you will feel stiff and tight. If you do experience pain, the medication will help you feel better.

Everyone responds differently to facial plastic surgery. Some patients feel great, if only because they were expecting to feel worse. After a face-lift, some patients have a tight feeling under their neck like a band of tissue is holding their neck in place. The cheek region is often numb, but this tends to pass and get better. Some people may have discomfort near their ears where the incisions are located. Patients who have had brow lifts may find that their eyes are a bit sensitive to light or feel slightly irritated, requiring drops.

Some Things to Remember as
You Move into the Recuperation Phase

- Expect to be tired. You've been through a lot, both physically and emotionally, and your body needs to rest from the whole experience.
- For at least the first twenty-four hours after surgery, make sure that you do not sign any important papers or make any significant decisions.
- Don't spend too much time looking in the mirror just yet. Newly placed stitches can be frightening at first glance, not to mention any bruising or swelling that may occur. I promise you will look better soon!

- If you had blepharoplasty (eye surgery), make sure you apply ice packs to your eyes every hour for the first thirty-six hours.
- Remember to keep your head elevated at all times for the first week or so (including while you sleep), as this decreases swelling and aids healing.
- Limit your activities for the first week to relaxing, staying at home, and being as comfortable as you possibly can. It's essential to have someone to care for you the first forty-eight hours—someone whom you can really count on to take care of everything without your guidance. We have found that friends or close relatives are best.
- *Follow your doctor's instructions.* This is critical, and failure to do so could result in complications or injury. Postpone driving until you are off medication and your surgeon gives you the okay. Pain medication can affect your ability to drive safely. Also, while driving you might have to make sharp turns, stop suddenly, or maybe even collide with something. Any of these can cause sutures to come loose, incisions to separate, bleeding resulting in hematomas, and many other problems.
- If you are going to experience complications related to bleeding, these generally occur within the first twenty-four to seventy-two hours. You need to be careful with coughing, sneezing, and vomiting. And definitely avoid all heavy lifting during this period.

CHAPTER FOURTEEN

The Healing Process

IN MY EXPERIENCE, WHAT MOST PEOPLE WANT after plastic surgery is instantaneous recovery. They think the process should be like getting a new hairstyle—you walk out of the doctor's office looking terrific and ready to resume your normal life. Unfortunately, it's just not like that. After any kind of surgical procedure, you need to heal and that takes *time*. The initial recovery process can last anywhere from a few days to a couple of weeks, depending on the type and extent of surgery. For many people, this period can be frustrating. But others just relax and enjoy it, which seems to me the more sensible approach.

Think of it as a forced vacation, one that is actually a lot more relaxing than most typical vacations. Traveling, even for fun, tends to be rather hectic. Run to the airport, get on the airplane, get off the airplane, take the taxicab or bus to the hotel, do a whirlwind of sightseeing and activities, and then go through the reverse to get home. Don't get me wrong. Travel can be stimulating and enjoyable, but it can also be wearing on your mind and body. By the time you return, you will typically need a few more days off to recuperate.

By contrast, during your post–plastic surgery "vacation," you have no choice but to take it easy. You can listen to music, read, listen to books on tape, watch television or videos, organize photos, or just sleep. It's completely unstructured time, and once they are able to let go, most people love it. Our lives are so structured most of the time that it's wonderful to have a break, and recuperation gives us an excuse to take it. Following is an overview of the typical recovery process.

THE FIRST FEW DAYS

You will probably see your doctor a day or so after surgery to have the dressing and drains removed. The doctor will also examine your sutures and check for any excessive swelling or bleeding as well as signs of infection, redness, or swelling. Your hair will likely be coarse and matted from the dressing and any drainage that occurred overnight. We usually ask our patients to try washing their hair the first day if they feel up to it, but you can wait until the second day if you prefer. Your hair should feel normal by the second or third washing. With the dressing and drains gone and your hair back to normal, you will begin to feel more like a human being.

Though I have not yet had a face-lift, patients usually tell me that their necks feel a bit tight at this stage. We ask them to pretend they are robots (at least in the early period), and to limit the motion of their face and neck. For example, if you need to see something to your right or left, turn your head and body together as one unit.

You will probably have some bruising and swelling. These tend to be worst around the fourth or fifth day before starting to improve. We've found that starting arnica a few days before surgery and continuing it after surgery helps decrease postoperative swelling. (Arnica is a supplement that you can buy at health food stores.)

Patients who have had mid-cheek lifts can develop swelling of the cheek area from lifting the cheek pad tissue. This swelling or fullness can take three to four months to resolve.

Follow-Up Visits

I usually see face-lift patients again on the fifth or sixth day to remove some of the sutures just in front of the ear. The behind-the-ear sutures are taken out after about ten days. Thereafter the follow-up visits stretch out at longer intervals until the recovery process is complete or nearly so. The number of follow-up visits will be determined by your doctor.

Follow-up visits are important for the doctor as well as the patient. The doctor needs to monitor closely the sutures, swelling, and changes in muscle and tissue. During these visits your doctor will also discuss such things as wound care and bandages, and what to expect with respect to swelling and bruising during the recovery period. Your doctor's office staff also serves as your reality check when it comes to questions about your recovery. Keep their phone number close by and call them with any concerns or questions that you might have. In particular, if you note any signs of possible infection or bleeding, call your doctor immediately. You are not doing them a favor by trying to "tough it out." The sooner any problems are dealt with, the better the outcome is likely to be.

Talking, Laughing, and Sleeping On Your Face

Every now and then I have a patient who is lively, talkative, and uses every muscle in his face to laugh. Although this can be a great social asset, it can create a challenge during the recovery process, too, because it is imperative to move your face as little as possible. I tell my patients to pretend they are ventriloquists and keep all talking and laughing to a bare minimum.

Also, if you're like many people, you often wake up with creases on your forehead, cheeks, and other parts of your face just from normal sleeping. It's critical to protect your face during the early stages of healing. Patients who have had mid-cheek lifts should be especially careful not to sleep on the sides of their face as this can cause sutures to loosen, possibly requiring a trip back to the operating room. A recliner will help you stay on your back and keep you from damaging your new look.

Post-Surgery Mood Swings

It is common for patients to feel happy and elated for the first two or three days following surgery. This is mostly a sort of euphoria that grows out of relief that the procedure is behind you. However, it is also common to experience a mood swing in the opposite direction once the initial thrill is gone. The person you see in the mirror will be a swollen and bruised stranger, and it will be tough to visualize the final results. You may feel like crying and not want anyone to see you (this typically includes friends and family). You may have doubts about whether you did the right thing by having the surgery and spending all that money.

Trust me, these thoughts are very common, and they will fade once the swelling and the bruising improve and the finished results become evident. In the meantime, you'll need the support and understanding of your family and friends during the early weeks. You may want to warn them ahead of time that you might turn into a real monster for a while. Your surgeon can also be helpful by responding to your questions and concerns—an important reason to pick a surgeon you feel comfortable talking to.

THE NEXT FEW WEEKS

Most people take a week to ten days off work to recuperate from a face-lift operation. For upper and lower lid blepharoplasty or eyelid surgery procedures, you would need about a week. For the upper lids only, four to five days may prove sufficient.

Although we recommend rest, rest, and more rest, many patients start conducting some business over the phone or Internet while recuperating during the first week. By the end of the week, most people are anxious to go back to work, if only to get out of the house.

For most of us, however, plastic surgery is a private matter, and we are concerned about what other people will think—especially our peers. So naturally we want to look perfect for our reentry into the world. If we were like most actors or actresses, we would take six months to a year off from public view after a face-lift or any other kind of facial surgery and not reappear until we looked great. Most people don't have that luxury, so you may still be a little rough around the edges when you return to the office. Using makeup to cover what's left of the bruising and artful hair arranging can help, along with a positive attitude to brush off any thoughtless or unkind comments.

As a plastic surgeon and also as a plastic surgery patient, I am familiar with the feelings that arise during the recovery process. Initially it can be difficult. You may feel like you're not the same person, as though part of you has been lost. However, in a surprisingly short time, you will learn to like your new, improved look. I can't tell you how many times my patients have told me, "I wish I'd done it sooner. My friends all tell me I look so good. I haven't told them why. I want to keep it my secret."

The Lumpy, Bumpy Skin Following a Face-Lift

After a face-lift, the skin on your cheeks and neck may have areas that feel like they are made of wood. Patients will come in for two- or three-week follow-up appointments and say, "Gee, Dr. Henry, what is this lumpy thing on my cheek?" I reassure them that it is part of the body's normal process of healing, and that collagen is being laid down to heal the area. Most patients are quite concerned about this, but with time the areas smooth out and look terrific. Sometimes we inject the area with a small amount of steroid, which helps the scar tissue to settle a bit more.

What About Scars?

For the most part, the incisions in front of the ear heal without much concern. Initially the scar will be quite pink, due to the collagen that is being deposited in the area as well as the blood supply.

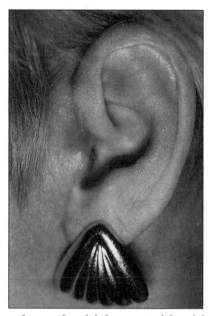

Figure 14.1 Three weeks post-face-lift for a typical face-lift incision.

During this time the incision can be easily covered by makeup. With time the blood supply to the incision site diminishes and the incision starts to fade.

The skin behind the ear is generally scalp skin and is thicker, requiring more healing time. Expect the incisions to be pink and noticeable for anywhere from three to eight months up to one year. Most people tend to grow their hair longer in this area or wear their hair down. Some patients use Scar Fade, a silicone product that helps the scar to smooth out and fade, or they use silastic sheeting to hide the incision until it fades naturally. (See Fig. 14.1.)

Exercise

Most patients are anxious to get back to exercising as soon as possible after surgery. Working out makes them feel good, and besides, they don't want to gain any weight from the enforced rest period. Like the rest of your life, exercise is something you have to ease back into after surgery. The first week you need to rest, period. After that, I recommend walking to my patients, as long as they do it in a safe environment and avoid rapid or sudden movements.

Do not do perform any heavy lifting for at least four to six weeks after your operation. That includes heavy bags of groceries or, for the parents among you, small children. You can sit down on the floor next to your child, or sit on the couch and let the child crawl to you. Being a mother myself, I understand how important mothering is, and I know that having surgery doesn't buy you time off from being a parent. Just don't pick your kids up for a while.

What About Sex?

One frequently asked question following plastic surgery is "When can I have sex?" I recommend that patients limit their exercise for at least four to six weeks, and this includes sex. Ultimately you want the best result possible, and that means following directions. So hold off on going back to the athletic club or engaging in sexual gymnastics for at least a month. After all, a complication could put you out of commission even longer.

Men and the Recovery Process

During the first day or so of the recovery phase, men have a tendency to act as though they have the worst case of flu in history. They all think they're going to die. But in most cases, this phase lasts only a day or so. After twenty-four hours, the guys turn the corner and look for something to do. Their minds get busy and in two or three days they're ready to get back to work. Men are for the most part task-oriented: Okay, now that that's taken care of, let's move on to whatever's next. Where a woman might be concerned about a last tiny remaining stitch, men may forget they have sutures in place and almost forget to have them taken out.

In general, the recovery process seems smoother for men than for women. From a plastic surgeon's standpoint, men tend to recuperate more quickly and require less follow-up and hand-holding than do women. Of course, there are exceptions to every rule, and I've seen women who recover very fast and men who take a long time. In general, though, men have an easier time of it.

THE FIRST YEAR

By three months after surgery, you're looking and feeling much better. The incision isn't so pink and the tight feeling under your neck is easing. If you had a mid-cheek lift, the swelling has pretty much resolved. Best of all, people are beginning to notice something different about you. They know you look better, but they can't quite say what's changed.

At six months, you are settling into your new look. The incision has faded considerably and you are more comfortable with everything including your decision to have the surgery in the first place.

Once you have healed and the swelling has dissipated, your surgeon will consider taking the "after" photographs. These are usually done in the same position and lighting as the first pictures to enable both of you to truly see the improvements. Some physicians use professional photographers.

At one year, you should be able to look back at your preoperative pictures and see a definite improvement. Your face feels more comfortable, softer, and more youthful, and you actually like looking in the mirror. Congratulations, you've made it! You made a decision to do something very special for yourself, you followed through, and now you get to reap the rewards. Enjoy your new look. You've earned it! (See Appendix 1: Procedures, Postoperative Restrictions, and Recovery Times.)

CHAPTER FIFTEEN

Postoperative Complications: How to Avoid Them and What to Do If They Occur

T HE DAY YOU SIGN UP FOR SURGERY with your plastic surgeon, you enter into an agreement between two people. Your surgeon agrees to provide you with a safe operation that protects your health while improving the effects of aging on your face. He has not agreed to make you look like someone you are not, or guaranteed that you will look twenty years younger. In return, you agree not only to pay for the doctor's services but to take responsibility for helping to protect your health and enable your surgery to be successful. This means keeping all of your preoperative and follow-up appointments and following all of your doctor's directions to the letter—both before and after surgery.

Complications from face-lifts are not common, but they can happen even to "perfect" plastic surgery patients who follow all instructions faithfully. This is rare, however. Complications tend to occur most often when patients don't follow postoperative instructions properly or ignore them altogether. Although the majority of complications are treatable and can be resolved without affecting the final result, they can be unpleasant, painful, and expensive. So it's best to avoid them if you possibly can.

I remember one patient who had a face-lift done just before Christmas one year. Late on the second night after her surgery, she decided she just had to do some more shopping, so she drove herself to the local mall and came home with two large bags full of purchases. About midnight she called my exchange to report that her face was hurting! By 2:00 A.M. I was back in the operating room evacuating a hematoma, a pool of blood and fluid that had collected under the skin flaps. Her final result was not affected, but it could have been if we had not been able to handle the problem quickly.

Generally speaking, whenever a complication occurs, a careful review of the days and hours leading up to the problem can pinpoint the main cause: The dog jumped up on me. I picked up a bag of groceries. I forgot to take my blood pressure medication. Two days before the operation I took an Alka-Seltzer and forgot to mention it. These types of complications are nearly always preventable. However, sometimes complications happen for reasons that are never determined. Both patients and surgeons must recognize that some risks are inherent in elective surgery, even though everything has been done to prevent problems from occurring.

Most complications fall into three broad categories: bleeding, infections, and scarring.

BLEEDING

In my practice, I see patients about two weeks prior to their operations. At this time I give them a booklet that describes the operation or operations that they will be having and provides detailed instructions for what they are to do—and not do—before and after surgery. The booklet includes a four-page list of all the medications patients are supposed to avoid in the two weeks before surgery. These include aspirin or aspirin-containing products and non-steroidal anti-inflammatories (NSAIDs) such as Advil or Motrin.

The reason that we tell patients to avoid these medications is because they adversely affect platelets in the blood. Platelets are the clot-forming cells that help stop bleeding should it occur. Because we can buy products such as aspirin or Advil over the counter (that is, without a prescription), we tend to think they are innocuous or somehow not "real" drugs. It is hard for people to understand how taking a couple of aspirin can cause bleeding problems a week or ten days later, but believe me, it can. If you forget, or if you just have such a bad headache or cramps that you decide you must take something, you must let your doctor know. They can perform a special blood test, called a bleeding time test, that measures how long it takes your blood to form a clot. If the bleeding time is short enough, surgery can proceed. If not, the safest thing to do is to postpone the operation until your bleeding time has improved.

Another common cause of bleeding problems is alcohol. This has been proven time and time again. It won't hurt you to skip that glass of wine with dinner or that after-work beer for two weeks before and at least a month after surgery. It could hurt you a lot if you don't.

High blood pressure can also lead to bleeding problems. If you are on medication for high blood pressure, make sure that you continue taking your medication both before and after your surgery unless your physician specifically says you do not need it.

Increased activity can also prove a culprit. I can remember one man who went water-skiing right after a rhinoplasty. He developed major bleeding from his nose that required three days in the hospital and a blood transfusion.

INFECTIONS

Infections are a risk with any type of surgery, occurring in perhaps 5 percent of all surgical cases. They are relatively rare in facial plastic surgery, which is probably due to routine use of antibiotics both before and after surgery.

The main symptoms of infection are redness, warmth, tenderness, and swelling, sometimes accompanied by a fever. After a facelift, infection can present as a hot boil on the surface of the skin, similar in appearance to a pimple. If this should happen, *do not* play with it. Instead, see your doctor as soon as you can. If it is an infection, he will prescribe additional antibiotics. In most cases, this should clear up the infection quickly. If you should develop an infection that is not responsive to oral antibiotics, your doctor may prescribe intravenous antibiotics. These can now be administered at home rather than in a hospital setting.

The best way to avoid infections is to follow your doctor's directions for wound care and take your full course of antibiotics. If you are immunocompromised for some reason, you will be more susceptible to infection. For this reason, people with immune system problems should avoid elective cosmetic surgery.

SCARRING

Scarring is a concern common to all operations. Scarring is unpredictable, but the best indicator of how much or how little you are likely to scar with cosmetic surgery is the way your skin has responded to past injuries—in other words, how much you have scarred in the past. Another factor is the location of the incision. Places where the skin is thicker, such as the scalp, will have more scarring than areas where the skin is thin, such as the face.

Incisions go through a series of transitions as they heal. About two weeks after surgery, they may look pretty good. By six weeks, as collagen builds up around a scar, it will look red, raised, lumpy, and bumpy. Don't be discouraged when this happens. It is a normal part of the healing process. By about three to six months, the scar will start to fade, and it will continue to improve over the next couple of years.

A scar that is raised, red, and noticeable can sometimes be improved with steroid injections, laser, or silastic gel sheeting. Often the best treatment is "Tincture of Time"—i.e., waiting it out.

Following are descriptions of the specific types of complications that can occur due to procedures discussed in this book.

COMPLICATIONS FOLLOWING FACE-LIFTS

In addition to the three most common complications, others specific to face-lifts include swelling, numbness, skin necrosis, loss of nerve function, hair loss or hairline changes, skin changes, chronic pain, and earlobe deformity.

Hematoma

A hematoma, or bleeding underneath a skin flap, is probably the worst complication that can occur following a face-lift. Although it is possible for a hematoma to happen to anyone, it is unlikely to occur if you follow instructions faithfully. The typical hematoma story is similar to that of the Christmas shopping lady earlier in this chapter.

The major symptom of a hematoma is swelling, which can occur on one or both sides of the face. You may also experience some difficulty breathing or swallowing. The skin may begin to look purplish, and sometimes blister. This is usually accompanied by a generally uncomfortable or "crummy" feeling.

If you experience any of these symptoms, call your doctor immediately. If you are alone (which by the way you should not be, especially during the early postoperative period), call an ambulance to take you to the nearest emergency room to meet your surgeon. Your surgeon will take you to the operating room, open one or both of your incisions, evacuate any fluid or blood that has accumulated,

and reclose the incisions. If you have sought help immediately after suspecting a hematoma, there is a good chance that your facial
skin will not suffer any major consequences. If you have waited a
significant period of time, however, there is a strong likelihood of
skin tissue necrosis. This is loss of tissue requiring close follow-up
with general wound care or possibly further revisionary surgery. Tissue necrosis can be worsened by smoking or exposure to secondhand smoke.

Scarring

The incision for a face-lift begins in front of the ear and travels behind the ear. For the most part, incisions in front of the ear heal
with minimal scarring. Because the skin behind the ear is thicker,
it tends to heal with more scarring. Occasionally, patients will develop a strong reaction to the sutures, which can cause widening of
the scar behind the ear. However, behind-the-ear scars can usually
be hidden by hair. The biggest risk for scarring is a history of smoking or exposure to secondhand smoke. Both can interfere with the
healing process.

Swelling

Virtually all patients experience some swelling after a face-lift. Most
surgeons recommend keeping your head elevated at all times during the healing process. I usually have my patients sleep on four to
six pillows for the first week, and reduce it to two to four the following week. I do not recommend using ice on the skin of the face
unless you have had an eyelid procedure. In this case, use ice packs
on the eyelids *only*.

Numbness

Numbness in the cheek area is normal following a face-lift. This is not worrisome and will improve, though it may take several weeks or even months. The scalp can also be quite numb, especially with a full brow lift. In rare cases the numbness may be permanent.

Skin Necrosis

Skin necrosis occurs when the skin tissue actually dies; it can happen as a result of an untreated hematoma. More often, it is caused by smoking or exposure to secondhand smoke. This is because nicotine constricts tiny blood vessels, resulting in a decrease in blood supply to the skin. Since blood is essential for healing, even a minor decrease in blood supply is dangerous. Be aware that nicotine patches can cause problems with wound healing after a face-lift.

The most common location for skin necrosis is the area right behind the ears. The affected area turns black and forms a hard scab that can take several weeks to heal. Some superficial scarring may be left as a result.

If you don't smoke, then don't worry about this problem. If you do smoke, quit at least a couple of weeks before you have face-lift surgery, and don't start up again until at least two weeks afterward (preferably never!).

Loss of Nerve Function

Though I have never seen a case of nerve function loss, I know that it does occur. The highest risk of nerve injury is in the SMAS or a subperiosteal face-lift. It is not the deep or superficial plane dissections but the middle plane of dissection that poses potential for nerve injury. During a deep SMAS dissection, the surgeon must work around the seventh facial nerve, which provides sensation and motor function to the facial muscles. If this nerve branch is damaged, the nerve function will be lost, in some cases permanently. Damage to smaller nerves is not as large a problem. This is because there is considerable "crossover" with regard to facial nerves. If a small branch nerve is damaged, several other neighborhood nerves will eventually take over the territory of the lost branch and provide function.

Some droopiness around the mouth is relatively common three to four days after a face-lift. This is usually due to swelling, or edema, of the facial nerve. The only treatment for this is time—anywhere from three or four months up to a year or even longer. Two other nerves that plastic surgeons need to watch out for are the frontalis branch and the marginal mandibular branch. The first allows you to raise your eyebrow, and the latter provides function to your lower lip. If either of these are gone after a face-lift, return of function is possible, but there may be a prolonged waiting period for swelling to improve.

If you are really worried about a problem with the SMAS dissection, then ask your surgeon to only perform a superficial face-lift in combination with a deep composite subperiosteal lift (a safe procedure that keeps you away from the nerves and provides a beautiful appearance to the mid-cheek area).

Hair Loss or Changes in Hairline Position

Hair loss behind the ear can occur with face-lifts, but this is rare. Brow lifts, however, require an incision that goes right along the hairline. Occasionally patients will lose some hair follicles along the incision line, particularly if their hair is thin to begin with. Sometimes we have patients use minoxidil (Rogaine) preoperatively, especially if they are quite worried about potential hair loss.

If the incision for the face-lift extends up into the temple area of the scalp, and/or into the hairline behind the ear, a patient is at risk for transient injury to the hair follicles. Regrowth of hair follicles usually takes place within fourteen weeks. The loss is usually noticed about two to three weeks postoperatively. Patients who smoke or have thin hair are at risk for having this problem.

Changes in hairline position can happen if the skin is pulled up too high. One telltale sign of a face-lift that you definitely want your surgeon to avoid is having the hair around the sideburn pulled up so much that a significant amount of forehead temporal skin is visible.

Skin Changes

Rarely, patients with darker skin, high risk of bruising, and/or overexposure to ultraviolet light may develop hyperpigmentation (dark pigmentation of the skin) in the area of the face-lift. This condition may require use of chemical peels or makeup following the procedure.

Chronic Pain

Most face-lift patients experience only minor, temporary discomfort, and skin sensation returns to normal within three to five months. However, in rare cases patients have reported chronic pain lasting a year or longer. Some patients complain that the operated areas get hot or red following exercise or for no apparent reason. While the reasons for these symptoms are unclear and there is no specific treatment, massage and ice packs may give some relief.

Earlobe Deformity

A "pixie ear" occurs when the earlobe is sewn to a point lower on the face than it was intended to be. This is relatively easy to correct and can be done by your surgeon under local anesthesia.

COMPLICATIONS FOLLOWING BROW LIFTS

As with face-lifts, the most serious complication that can occur with a brow lift is a hematoma, which can lead to tissue loss. The most common complication is itching of the forehead or scalp, which can last for several months. In rare cases, patients may experience weakness or paralysis on one or both sides of the forehead following a brow lift. This usually goes away within a few months, although in some cases it may be permanent. Numbness is also common with standard brow lifts and may take several months to resolve. It is less likely, though still possible, with endoscopic lifts.

Although it is not common, partial removal of the muscles that cause frowning or forehead wrinkles may leave small, barely noticeable depressions in the skin of the forehead.

COMPLICATIONS FOLLOWING BLEPHAROPLASTY

As with face-lifts, the primary complications that can occur following blepharoplasty are bleeding, infection, and scarring. A number of patients develop dry eyes, requiring frequent use of eye drops for a few months. Tiny cysts sometimes form along the incision lines. These often clear up by themselves, or the surgeon can "pick them out" with a needle tip.

Less common complications include inadequate resection of fatty tissue and excess skin that was not excised in the initial operation. These can be revised with a second operation. The opposite problem, removal of too much skin, can lead to an inability to close the upper eyelids; in these cases a skin graft may be needed to repair the lids. In rare cases, upper eyelid surgery may damage the mechanism that supports and lifts the upper eyelid, causing the eyelid to sag. This may require further surgery.

With lower lid surgery, some people experience sagging of the eyelids due to temporary or long-term loss of the muscle's nerve function. The nerve function usually returns within several days to weeks. Supporting the eyelid with tape and upward massage usually helps, and few patients require further surgery. More commonly, removal of too much fat can leave hollows under the eyes.

Cornea injuries due to exposure can occur but are rare, as is keratitis, a problem with drainage due to swelling. Vision loss is an extremely rare complication and is caused by bleeding within the orbit around the eye.

If for any reason after a blepharoplasty you develop tightness around your eyelids and difficulty with your vision, you need to tell your plastic surgeon immediately.

COMPLICATIONS FOLLOWING IMPLANTS

In addition to infection, bleeding, and scarring, complications that can occur with implants include nerve injury and asymmetry. Permanent nerve damage is rare. However, temporary numbness in the area of the implant is common; in some cases slight numbness may be permanent. Slight drooping and stiffness of the lower lip and chin commonly occur with chin implants. These usually subside in a few weeks without treatment.

Occasionally implants may shift out of position either soon after surgery or within several months. This is usually caused by some sort of trauma, such as a blow to the face, and may require surgery to reposition the implant.

Many implants are made of silicone rubber. Although silicone has not been implicated in any diseases and has been used in many types of implants, its use is under investigation.

If for any reason an implant needs to be removed, it should not be replaced for at least two months.

COMPLICATIONS
FOLLOWING BOTOX INJECTIONS

Most people experience some redness, swelling, and headaches during the first week or so after treatment. A small percentage have temporary drooping of their eyelids, which can last for several months.

Because antibiotics can increase the potency of Botox, be sure to tell your doctor if you are taking any.

COMPLICATIONS
FOLLOWING COLLAGEN INJECTIONS

The most common complications following collagen injections are allergy and infection, both of which are rare. Allergy problems can be avoided by doing a patch test prior to the injections.

COMPLICATIONS FOLLOWING FAT TRANSFERS

The primary complication that can occur with fat implants is fat being reabsorbed into the body and the effect being lost. Experience has shown that subsequent fat transfers tend to last longer. Some patients have lumpiness under the skin that can be felt and, more rarely, becomes visible. Massage and, of course, time generally resolve this problem.

COMPLICATIONS FOLLOWING LASER RESURFACING

Complications that can occur with laser resurfacing include scarring, skin discoloration, prolonged redness, herpes skin infections, cysts, and incomplete removal of wrinkles or irregularities.

Scarring

Scarring can occur when resurfacing goes into the dermis rather than staying on the top layers of the skin. The pulsed CO_2 lasers are so precise that this happens only rarely, and when it does, it is generally confined to small areas. Scarring that does occur can be treated with pressure and injected steroids, but in most cases time is the best healer.

Skin Discoloration

In rare cases, laser resurfacing can cause the skin to become darker (hyperpigmentation). Even more rarely, damage to the pigment cells can cause the skin to become lighter (hypopigmentation). The change, if any, is usually mild.

Prolonged Redness

Once the initial healing period has passed, the skin will generally be red or pink; this gradually fades over the following two to six months. If the redness persists, it can be treated with a bleaching agent and Retin-A.

Herpes Skin Infections

Any skin resurfacing method can stir up dormant herpes infections. This can occur regardless of whether you have had previous herpes outbreaks. In severe cases, the sores can spread and cause permanent scars. The best treatment for herpes outbreaks is prevention. For this reason, most surgeons have patients take an antiherpes agent such as acyclovir before the resurfacing procedure.

Cysts

Small pinpoint white cysts called milia may form on the surface of the skin following laser resurfacing, most commonly around the eyes. These generally go away on their own, or the surgeon can remove them with a needle during a simple in-office procedure.

Incomplete Removal of Wrinkles or Irregularities

If you have deep wrinkles, one treatment may not be enough to resolve them because going too deeply would create a risk of scarring. Also some growths, birthmarks, and tattoos may respond partially or not at all to laser resurfacing. Additional laser treatments or other procedures may be required to achieve the desired results.

CHAPTER SIXTEEN

What Will It Cost and How Will I Pay for It?

WHEN YOU CONSIDER HAVING COSMETIC SURGERY, a host of questions will go through your mind. Is it really a good idea? Is it for me? Do I have realistic expectations? When can I schedule it? Can I find someone to help me with the kids? And then there is the big one: Can I really afford to do this?

As plastic surgery has become more and more popular among the general population (that is, those of us who are not yet or never will be movie stars, news anchors, or jet-setters), the affordability factor has become a major concern. However, in the past few years plastic surgery has become increasingly affordable. Some people even view it as a business expense. Especially for people who are in the public eye, appearance can be a major factor in landing or keeping a job.

A recent poll indicated that the average annual income of plastic surgery patients was between $30,000 and $35,000 a year — considerably less than the annual rent on the average Beverly Hills mansion. Obviously plastic surgery isn't just for the rich and famous anymore. Waitresses, construction workers, school teachers, secretaries, real estate agents, homemakers, salespeople — my patients come from just about every background and occupation you can think of. Like so many other things, it's generally a matter of where there's a will, there's a way. If you want it badly enough, you will find a way to come up with the money.

Not that plastic surgery is cheap. For a basic face-lift you can plan on spending at least $5,000. Start adding other procedures such as

a brow lift or laser resurfacing and the total can go up to $15,000 or
more. (Appendix 2 shows fee ranges for all of the procedures discussed in this book.) Fees vary, of course, among individual physicians and different parts of the country. Generally where the cost of
living is higher, fees will be, too. You would pay more in New York,
for example, than in Kansas City or Des Moines.

Members of the American Society of Plastic Surgeons have their
fees monitored by the organization. The rule is that members cannot charge exorbitant fees for their work. In practice, this means that
the fees should be similar to what is charged by other physicians in
the same geographic area. If you live in Los Angeles, for example,
where a number of surgeons commonly work on movie stars, the
standard fees are going to be higher than they would be in, say, St.
Louis. In addition to monitoring fees, the ASPRS also sets standards
for advertising and educational requirements.

In addition to the surgeon's fees, you must also consider all of the
other costs involved. These include fees for the use of the operating
room in the hospital, surgery center, or doctor's office; the fee for
the anesthesiologist and any assisting physicians; and the cost of
medications. Since cosmetic surgery is considered elective in the
vast majority of cases, you will probably not be able to rely on insurance to defray or cover any part of these costs.

If you need to hire someone to care for you the first day or you
are going to a retreat or recovery center, you will have to pay for that
as well. Then there is the cost of time off from work, child care, pet
boarding, and so on. Make sure that you include all of these when
you are working out how to pay for your surgery or you could be in
for some unpleasant surprises.

WHEN IS A BARGAIN NOT A BARGAIN?

When it comes to having someone make permanent changes to
your face, not to mention doing things that could have a major effect on your health, what seems like a good deal may in fact turn

out to be very bad indeed. If a patient coordinator—or, worse, a doctor—quotes you a price that seems low, a red flag should go up immediately. You should be especially wary if the doctor himself is the one providing the price quotes. Your surgeon should be focusing on you and the surgical procedures she will be performing, not on what she expects to earn.

Some surgeons tend to resort to "bargain basement prices" when business is slow on the theory that business will pick up and they can make up the difference in volume. Take this as a friendly warning. In plastic surgery, you usually get what you pay for, so caution is advised.

PAYMENT OPTIONS

Most plastic surgeons have a patient coordinator or other staff person whose role is to discuss fees and financial arrangements. This is usually done at the time of the initial consultation or soon thereafter.

The vast majority of plastic surgeons require full payment prior to the surgery date, usually by the time of the pre-op appointment. Other fees related to the surgery, such as the fee for the operating room (if done in the hospital) and the fee for the anesthesiologist, are usually paid on the day of the operation.

Fees can be paid by check, credit card, or, of course, cash. Many doctors are now able to offer their patients financing through independent finance companies. Your doctor's patient coordinator can tell you if this is an option. If you choose this option, you will have to pass a credit check and be approved for the loan. If you are approved, you will be making monthly payments on both the principal and interest for the next several years just as you would for your mortgage or your car. This form of payment has made plastic surgery more feasible for many patients who formerly were unable to afford it.

CHAPTER SEVENTEEN

A Face-Lift Journal

A S I SEE IT, A FACE-LIFT IS A PROCESS—it unfolds in stages. From the decision to choose surgery, to the final result, it is a personal journey. I believe you take out of the process exactly what you put into it. Plastic surgery is a wonderful tool for enhancing your spirit, self-image, and self-confidence. But it is not a panacea for life's problems, and it does not change you into a different person at the core level.

I felt I was a good candidate for plastic surgery, in that I fit the criteria, and I was losing self-confidence because my inside did not match my outside. I believe I was dealt a hand of premature aging, which was especially difficult because until that time (age thirty-nine) I always looked very youthful.

And so my journey began through what I consider a well-researched, intelligent series of choices, from selecting a doctor to the final result. I can't emphasize enough the importance of choosing a doctor who not only has great communication skills, excellent technical skills, a natural sense of artistry, and recognized certification, but who is a caring individual, too. After a careful search that started by asking friends and following up their recommendations, I found what I was looking for in Dr. Kimberly Henry.

Having gotten this far, my fear of surgery gave way to excitement. After the initial doctor-patient consultation, I realized that if I was to make this into a positive experience, it was essential to follow the instructions given to me by Dr. Henry and her staff. I was given a folder with detailed information about the whole process, which I really appreciated, and guidance on how to prepare for the operation.

Taking good care of myself in the pre-surgery stage was important to me. I felt it would give me more strength and confidence and, of course, aid in the healing process. I addressed this by following an exercise program, eating a well-balanced diet, practicing stress management techniques, getting plenty of rest, and generally being mindful of increasing my level of self-care. Not that I followed it perfectly, of course, but focusing in that direction really helped.

I also made sure my home was prepared so that my return from surgery would be as comfortable as possible. I went all out to create a nurturing, healing environment: crackers and 7-Up for the first day at home, fresh flowers to nourish my spirit, magazines with great photographs, uplifting videos, and anything else I could think of to make things comfy and inviting. I knew the postoperative period would amount to a serious retreat, and that I would need quiet and rest to heal. I placed a box by the bed filled with everything I might need including pain medication, arnica (a natural cream for bruising), and some other items Dr. Henry had given me to aid in the healing process. I also asked a friend who had previously had a face-lift herself to be there with me for the first couple of days—a good move!

The morning of surgery, I felt prepared and mostly on top of it. An edge of anxiety was definitely there—but so was the excitement. My husband drove me to the office the first thing in the morning. He was supportive and that helped a great deal. I arrived to find a nurturing staff, which I really appreciated, because every bit of warmth helps at that point. I met the anesthesiologist, who was very professional and kind. I also had the opportunity to speak with Dr. Henry for a brief time before the surgery, which was reassuring. We went over my expectations one more time (as if she needed to hear it again—I had written a detailed outline for her as well). Again, I felt both anxiety and excitement, side-by-side.

The next thing I knew I was waking up in a fog. This is when the staff is really an important part of the team, and Dr. Henry's staff was the best. I knew that I was in good hands and felt ready to surrender to the process ahead of me. My head was bandaged with only my face exposed. When he saw me, my husband immediately nicknamed me the "English Patient." A sense of humor definitely helps at that time! I felt quite vulnerable, but at the same time I knew I was in good loving hands. And I was indeed a pumpkin head!

This was when I needed to work on my mind. I kept telling myself, "Don't give in to negative thoughts and don't panic. This is all temporary." Despite the bandages and the fogginess, I felt a sense of confidence, though not comfort by any stretch. The discomfort wasn't really pain so much (the pain was there, but quite tolerable with the medication). It was more an overall feeling of acute sensitivity. I continued to remind myself that what I was experiencing was perfectly normal, and I tried to relax.

I got home to a well-prepared environment and loving care. I did nothing that first day but rest, rest, rest. My stomach was upset from the surgery, so I sipped 7-Up and nibbled soda crackers. I knew that once I made it through the first night, I would be well on my way toward healing. (I did remind myself often to keep a positive attitude. My condition was temporary.) The next day the bandages came off, and there was nothing left to do but heal. There was something reassuring about having the actual surgery behind me and moving on to the next stage.

The swelling and bruising started early on, almost as soon as I got home. The swelling was not entirely even. Luckily I had read enough to expect that, so I was not terribly concerned to discover that my eyes were not exactly the same size. The bruising soon spread and deepened to a dark purplish color (later it faded to a light yellowish tint— hurray for makeup!). In essence, I was a sight! But the pain faded fairly quickly, giving way to a general, but tolerable, sensation of discomfort.

As the days went by, the change became dramatic. It was truly thrilling! I could see this face peering back at me in the mirror, and it was youthful (at least ten years younger looking) and refreshed. I knew that it was still important to stay rested and quiet. Even though I was feeling more energetic, I still had a significant amount of healing left.

I also knew that a number of people go through a brief depression following surgery. I can't say I didn't have my moments, but overall I could not have been happier. This was just the change that I had been looking for. I was still me, but I was more youthful looking and refreshed. Having a face-lift was a gift to myself to bring more quality to my life. It was not intended to have me look like someone else. It was intended to help me hit my personal best.

So the days passed and I had a retreat from the world for about two and a half weeks. I do admit I was a little daunted at the prospect of going back to my life and carrying on as usual. Would other people comment? Amazingly enough, they did, but the comments were all along the lines of "You look so rested and refreshed." I felt positively buoyant! As I stated earlier, having plastic surgery does not take away life's problems. For me, however, it lifted my spirit and allowed me to bring forth my true self and enjoy life more fully.

It is nearly one year since my face-lift surgery, and I must say I hold a deep appreciation and respect for Dr. Kimberly Henry and her staff. Dr. Henry's professionalism and artistry were impeccable. Like everyone, I have my normal share of ups and downs, but in spite of it all, the face-lift from beginning to end was my midlife gift to myself. It has enhanced my connection to myself, to the world, and to life.

SUSAN

Appendixes

Appendix 1 Procedures, Postoperative Restrictions, and Recovery Times

Procedure	Postoperative Pain/Discomfort	Postoperative Restrictions	Initial Recovery Period	Final Results Visible
Blepharoplasty Upper lid	Minimal Oral pain meds for 1–2 days	Minimal eyestrain (TV, computer) No heavy lifting for 4–6 weeks No aerobics for 4–6 weeks Eyedrops required for 3–4 months for patients with dry eyes	4–5 days	2–3-weeks
Lower lid	Minimal Oral pain meds for 1–2 days	No heavy lifting for 4–6 weeks No aerobics for 4–6 weeks	4–7 days	2–3 weeks (but may take longer with lower lids) up to 3–4 months
Botox injections	Minimal postinjection pain	Limit contact use for 7–10 days postoperatively No headstands Don't massage the area near injection site	1–2 hours May have mild headache	4 days to 2 weeks to see full paralysis
Brow lift Standard	Headache for 1–2 days	No heavy lifting for 4–6 weeks No aerobics for 4–6 weeks No hair color treatments for 3 weeks Must wash hair daily beginning second day post-op to keep area clean	5–7 days	Immediate up to 6 weeks

Procedure	Discomfort	Restrictions		
Endoscopic	Headache for 1–2 days	No heavy lifting for 4–6 weeks No aerobics for 4–6 weeks No hair color for 3 weeks Wash hair daily	5–7 days	Immediate up to 6 weeks
Cheek implants	Minimal Swelling as though you had wisdom teeth removed Can last for 3 weeks	Must stay on liquid/soft diet for 7–10 days Minimal laughing, talking, smiling	5–7 days	3 months
Chin implant	Minimal Moderate aching in chin easily relieved	Must stay on liquid/soft diet for 7–10 days Minimal laughing, talking, smiling	5–7 days	3 months Expect swelling for 10 days
Collagen injections	Minimal	Limit massage in the area of injection, unless told to do so	14 hours	24 hours Some lumpiness Will smooth out with time
Face-lift	Minimal for most patients	Keep head elevated No exercise for 1–2 weeks No heavy lifting for 4–6 weeks No aerobics for 4–6 weeks	1–2 weeks	Acceptable in 5–6 weeks 10–12 months for complete settling
Fat injections	Minimal	No manipulation of injected area No heavy lifting for 4–6 weeks No aerobics for 4–6 weeks	2–3 days	3 weeks to 3 months

Continued overleaf

Appendix 1 Procedures, Postoperative Restrictions, and Recovery Times, *continued*

Procedure	Postoperative Pain/Discomfort	Postoperative Restrictions	Initial Recovery Period	Final Results Visible
Full-face laser skin resurfacing	First 24 hours okay; 2–5 days uncomfortable "stinging," similar to a bad sunburn	No heavy lifting for 10 days No sun exposure No picking at skin	8–10 days	See nice improvement in 3–6 weeks Up to 4 months for redness to subside
Lip augmentation	Minimal	No heavy lifting for 4–6 weeks No aerobics for 4–6 weeks	3–7 days	7 days to 8 weeks Swelling may be present for 7 days. AlloDerm swelling may last 8 weeks
Mid-cheek lift	Minimal	Limit movement of face, including talking, laughing, yawning No heavy lifting for 4–6 weeks No aerobics for 4–6 weeks	7–10 days	3–4 months
Mini face-lift	Minimal	Limit neck motion No heavy lifting for 4–6 weeks No aerobics for 4–6 weeks	5–7 days	2–3 weeks

| *Neck liposuction/ microsuction* | Almost none | No heavy lifting for 4–6 weeks
No aerobics for 4–6 weeks
Must wear garment to achieve an excellent result in contour— 24 hours/day for first 7 days, then at least 12 hours/day for 4–6 weeks | 3–5 days | 3–6 months |

Appendix 2 Average Fees and Related Costs for Procedures

Procedure	Surgeon's Fees (National Average)	Duration of Procedure	Average Operating Room Fee			Anesthesia Cost
			In-Office	Surgery Center	Hospital	
Blepharoplasty						
Upper lid	$1,750–$2,200	1 hour	$400–$850	$1,000	$1,200	$250/hour
Lower lid	$2,000–$2,500	1 hour, 15 min.	$400–$850	$1,000	$1,200	$250/hour
Botox injections	$475–$900	30 seconds	N/A	N/A	N/A	N/A
Brow lift						
Standard	$3,000–$5,000	2–3 hours	$850	$1,500	$1,500	$250/hour
Endoscopic	$2,600–$4,200	45 min.–3 hours	$1,000	$1,400	$1,600	$250/hour
Cheek implants	$2,000–$4,000	1–2 hours	$850	$850	$1,000	$250/hour
Chin implant	$2,000–$3,000	1–1 1/2 hours	$850	$850	$1,000	$250/hour
Collagen injections	$275–$450	15 min.	N/A	N/A	N/A	Local, included in fee
Face-lift	$4,800–$10,000	4–6 hours	$1,600	$2,000	$3,000	$250/hour
Fat injections	$1,500–$4,500	1–3 hours	$650–$850	$850	$1,200	$250/hour
Full-face laser skin resurfacing	$3,000–$6,000	1–2 hours	$350	$650	$1,000	$250/hour
Lip augmentation	$2,000–$4,000	1 hour	N/A	N/A	N/A	Local, included in fee
Mid-cheek lift	$3,000–$4,500	2 hours	$850	$1,200	$1,500	$250/hour
Mini face-lift	$2,000–$3,000	1–2 hours	$650	$1,000	$1,000	$250/hour
Neck liposuction/ microsuction	$2,000	1 hour	$650	$1,000	$1,000	$250/hour

Resources

American Society of Plastic
  Surgeons
444 E. Algonquin Road
Arlington Heights, IL 60005
Phone: (847) 228-9000
1-800-635-0635

American Board of Plastic
  Surgery
Steve Penn Center, Suite 400
35 Market Street
Philadelphia, PA 19103
Phone: (215) 587-9322

American Society for Aesthetic
  Plastic Surgeons, Inc.
444 E. Algonquin Road
Arlington Heights, IL 60005
Phone: (847) 228-99274

The American Medical
  Association
515 North State Street
Chicago, IL 60610
Phone: (312) 464-5000

The American Academy of
  Facial Plastic and
  Reconstructive Surgery
1101 Vermont Avenue, N.W.
Suite 404, Dept. MC
Washington, D.C. 20005
Phone: 1-800-332-3223

*Also contact your local medical
society and hospitals and
medical centers in your area.*

Index